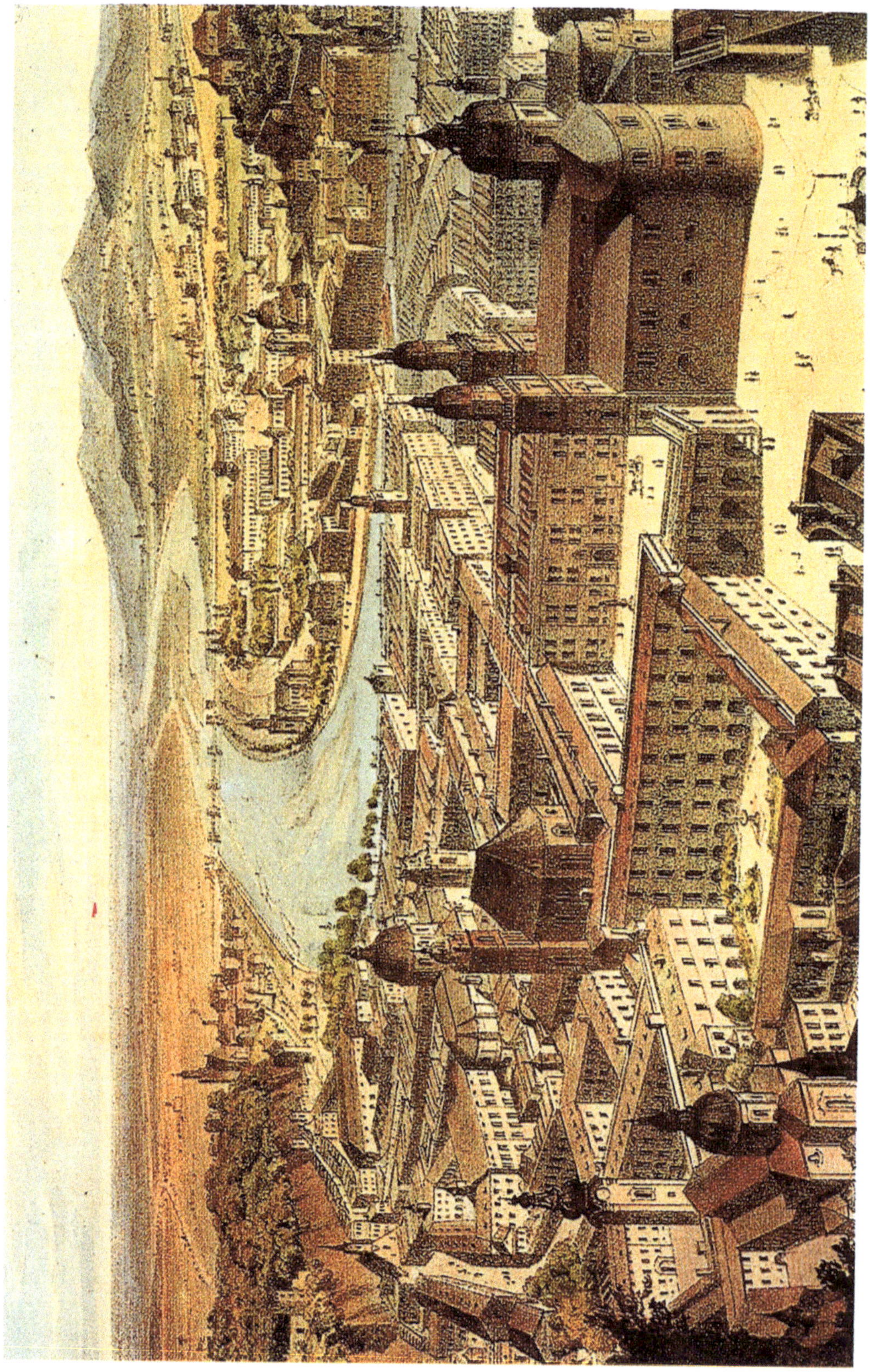

Alec Eden

The Search for Christian Doppler

Springer-Verlag Wien GmbH

Prof. Alec Eden
The Christian Doppler Foundation
Schwarzstrasse 44, A-5020 Salzburg, Austria

Originally published by Springer-Verlag Wien New York in 1992

Printed on acid-free paper

With 27 partly colored Figures

Frontispiece: Salzburg at the time of Christian Doppler (ca. 1840)
From a coloured lithograph by Leopold Rottmann after Georg Pezolt. The house in which Doppler was born is on the far bank of the River Salzach and is indicated by the tip of the small square tower of the City Hall on the near side, slightly to the right of the centre of the picture.

Cover design: T. Erben, Wien

Library of Congress Cataloging-in-Publication Data.

Eden, Alec, 1935— . The Search for Christian Doppler / Alec Eden. p. cm. Includes index. ISBN 978-3-7091-7378-7 ISBN 978-3-7091-6677-2 (eBook)
DOI 10.1007/978-3-7091-6677-2
1. Doppler, Christian, 1803—1853. 2. Physicists — Austria — Biography. I. Title. QC16.D7E34 1992. 530'.092—dc20. [B]. 92-16814

ISBN 978-3-7091-7378-7

This book is dedicated to my daughter, Guinevere,
and other young scientists of her generation
at the threshold of an exciting career

Foreword

It is now 150 years ago, on 25th May 1842, that the son of a Salzburg stonemason presented a scientific work "On the coloured light of the double stars and certain other heavenly bodies" at a meeting of the Royal Bohemian Society of Sciences held in Prague. Christian Andreas Doppler, then professor at the Prague Technical Institute, set a milestone in scientific history in the meeting room of the Royal Society in the Charles University, just a few meters from the National Theatre where another genius from Salzburg, Wolfgang Amadeus Mozart, had celebrated his musical triumph with the première of his opera *Don Giovanni* fifty-five years earlier.

Doppler's lecture set out in brilliant simplicity what we now call the Doppler principle, which since has found numerous uses in astronomy, which was of primary interest to Christian Doppler. In addition, it has found countless practical applications in physics, navigation, aeronautics, geodesy, medicine, science and technology. In medicine alone, Doppler sonography is now an established diagnostic procedure in the fields of childbirth, cardiology and diseases of the blood vessels, neurology, neurosurgery and vascular surgery, and is continually finding new medical applications in today's world of high technology.

It is only recently that we have been able to inform ourselves about the life and work of Christian Doppler, with the publication of Professor Alec Eden's first biographical portrait of the Salzburg physicist in 1988, the year in which he was appointed to the Presidency of the Christian Doppler Foundation in the city of Doppler's birth. It is in keeping with the objectives of this Foundation that Professor Eden is not only well known for his historic researches into Doppler's works, but also for the most recent developments of Doppler sonography in the prevention and treatment of stroke and other diseases of the brain.

This new book, published to commemorate the 150th anniversary of the discovery of the Doppler principle in Prague, contains much new information and gives us a fascinating insight into the life of the great scientist.

Dr. Hans Katschthaler
Governor of the State of Salzburg

Author's Acknowledgements

Unfortunately it is not possible here to thank numerous people who have given me willing and unstinting help in my search for Christian Doppler. This expression of gratitude to those who have been my main support at the various stations in Christian Doppler's life should be considered also as representing the countless others who have contributed even small stones to the mosaic.

In Salzburg special thanks are due to the late Ludwig Gollnacker, master stonemason in Himmelreich and his family, Bartholomäus Reischl for his painstaking and excellently documented geneological research in the parish of Wals, Liselotte Jetzelsberger-Lanik for her repeated kind hospitality in Doppler's house, as well as Professor Gunther Ladurner and Dr. Peter Mittermayr for their untiring efforts in the activities of the Christian Doppler Foundation. Memories of the enthusiasm of the first director of the Foundation, Karl Färbinger whose sudden death in 1990 robbed us of a dedicated Doppler researcher, have also given me great encouragement to complete this work. I have also been very fortunate to receive the fullest support from the Salzburg State Government and its two successive Governors, Dr. Wilfried Haslauer and Dr. Hans Katschthaler, to whom I am especially grateful for their personal engagement.

In Vienna the cooperation of Dr. Augusta Dick and Dr. Wolfgang Kerber, Director of the Central Library for Physics at the University of Vienna, has been especially valuable as has that of Professor Helmut Grössing and Dr. Peter Schuster, fellow searchers for Christian Doppler. To Christian Doppler's great granddaughter, Dorothea Merstallinger, special thanks are due for the many fascinating details on the life of her relatives.

In Prague I am above all greatful to President Vaclav Havel and his fellow "dissidents" in the struggle for freedom, without which proper research is impossible. It has been a pleasure to receive the kind cooperation of Professor Otto Wichterle, President of the Czechoslovakian Academy of Sciences, and Dr. Jindřich Schwippel who carefully safeguards the archives of the successor to the Royal Bohemian Society of Sciences. Professor Jan Havránek, Director of the Charles University Archives, and Dr. Štefan Zajac of the Faculty of Mathematics and Physics at that historic university have been sources of much valuable information concerning Doppler's time in the Golden City, as has Dr. Ivan Štoll of the Czech Technical University, where Doppler taught. Dr. Karl Peterlik, Austrian Ambassador in Prague, has been a gracious host and a wonderful organiser of contacts in the somewhat chaotic months following the "velvet revolution".

In Doppler's final resting place of Venice, it has been my pleasure to receive the warm hospitality of the Mayor, Dr. Antonio Casselatti and the kind help of Dr. Alessandro Franchini of the Venetian Institute for Science, Letters & Arts, and Dr. Sergio Barizza of the Municipal Historical Archives. My thanks are due to them and to Professor Diego Fontanari and his colleague Dr. Adriano Campioni at the Hospital of *Santi Giovanni e Paolo*, who together with their journalist friend, Riccardo Vianello, have been of great help in documenting Doppler's last days.

Considerable support and encouragement for the writing of this book has also been obtained from the many letters from readers of my previous biographical sketch of Doppler, publishing in 1988. A cardiologist in Teheran, who uses Doppler echocardiography daily in his practice, quoted an ancient Chinese philosopher: "The one who drinks water should think of he who has dug the well."

Thanks are also due to Brenda Shanks and Richard Craven for their help in the proof reading of the manuscripts, and to the staff of Springer-Verlag for their friendly cooperation in ensuring that this book should appear on the 150th anniversary of Doppler's famous work.

Finally, I should like to thank my family for their understanding and support of my search for Christian Doppler, especially my son Magnus who took over the difficult task of translating his famous work into English.

To all, and the many others, thank you.

Salzburg, Spring 1992 Alec Eden

Contents

List of Illustrations

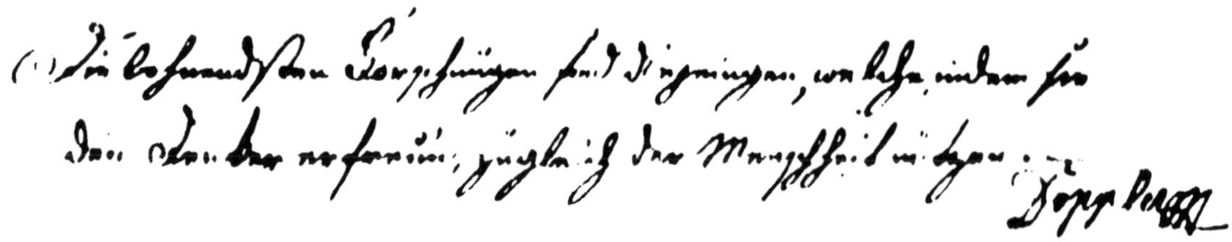

„Die lohnendsten Forschungen sind diejenigen, welche in dem sie den Denker erfreu'n, zugleich der Menschheit nützen."

Doppler

"The most rewarding researches are those which, inasmuch as they are a joy to the thinker, are at the same time of benefit to mankind."

Doppler

Christian Andreas Doppler
This daguerreotype was probably made by Wilhelm Horn in Prague, possibly at the same time in 1844 as he made the family portrait which appears on page 46. At this time Doppler was very much engaged in work on measuring instruments (diastemometer, omatogoniometer) on which he published several papers the following year. It is likely that the instrument pictured beside him is one of these inventions.

(Original in Museum Carolino Augusteum, Salzburg)

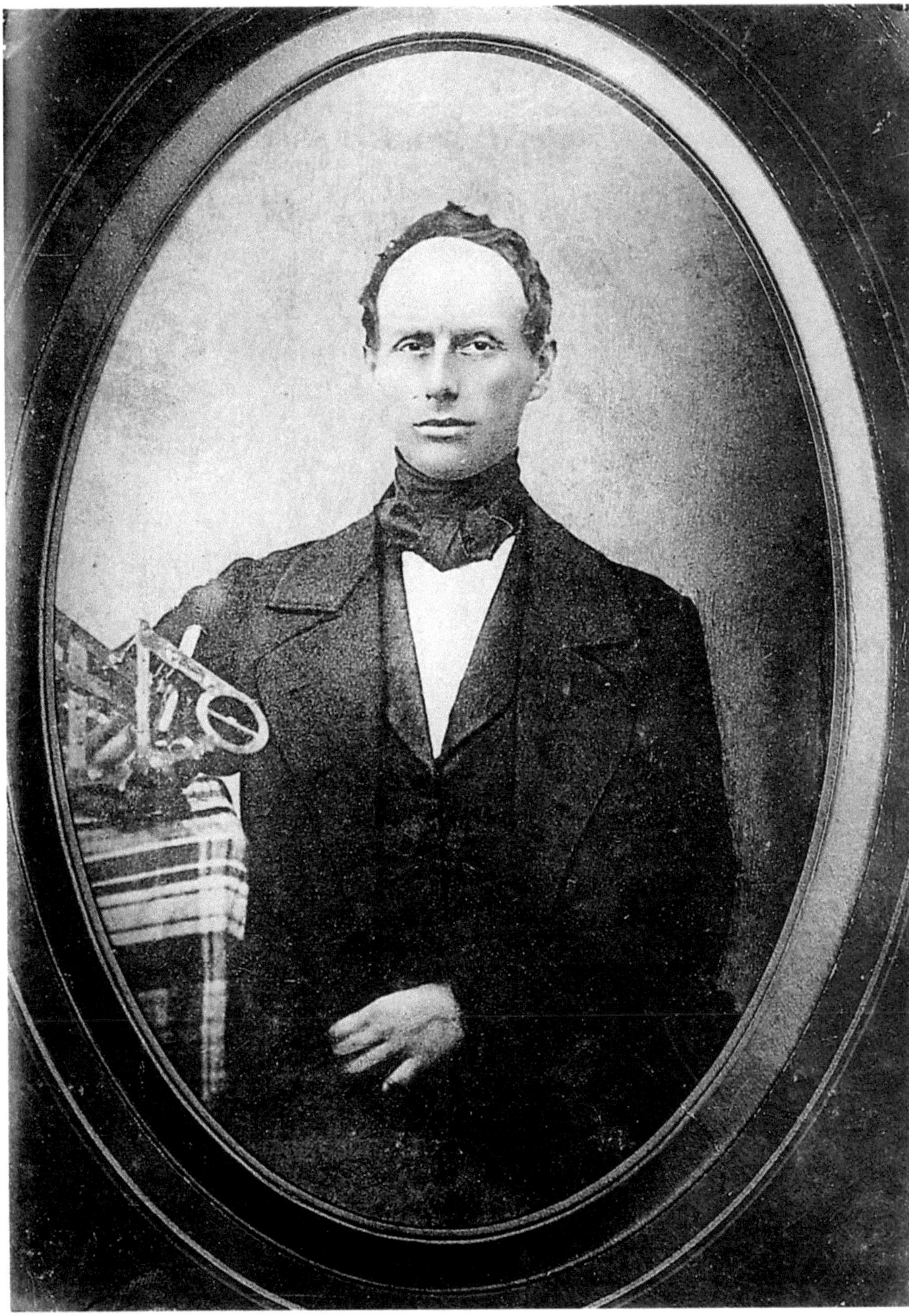

The Search for Christian Doppler

A glance at my watch told me it was three o'clock. Another night almost completely taken up with work on this series of lectures. The first one — the really important one — was only a few short weeks away. Important for me because it was my first as visiting professor at a major American university, the prestigious Health Sciences Center of the University of Texas at Dallas — and in the Department of Neurosurgery. It was here in 1963 that the dying President John F. Kennedy was brought in a last vain attempt to save his life. It was here that my host professor and Chairman of the Department, Dr. Kemp Clark, then a young resident later to become President of the World Federation of Neurosurgery, told Jacqueline Kennedy that her husband — the most powerful man in the world — was dead (62).

Lecturing to neurosurgeons — even the most famous — did not worry me too much, although I had only worked in my own innovative area of this speciality for about five years. But Kemp Clark had told me that this first lecture would be relayed by closed-circuit television to every medical school in Texas. I forget how many viewers he told me I would have, but for me my Dallas debut assumed the proportions of the soap opera of the same name. A glance through my lecture notes reassured me that what I had to convey to these viewers of the neurosurgical "Dallas" would have as great an impact as even the most exciting episode of its lay counterpart.

My presentation would inform them how Doppler sonography, the application of ultrasound in combination with the Doppler principle, could tell them whether the blood was flowing adequately in any one of the countless blood vessels in the human brain. The miniaturised transducers that had been developed by our research team could be placed on the arteries during the operation to reassure them that the tiny blood vessels they had just sewn together under the operating microscope were fulfilling their function as a blood-supplying bypass to an oxygen starved area of the brain. Or that the life threatening aneurysm had been made harmless by being clipped off, without impairing flow in the blood vessel itself. These were sequelae that until now were evident only after the skull had been closed and the operation completed. Thanks to the clinical researches of Professor Joachim Gilsbach and his colleagues at the University Hospital at Freiburg in Germany, working together with Dr. Dominique Cathignol in France and ourselves, this use of Doppler sonography was able to reduce the death rate of such neurosurgical interventions from about 5 % to zero.

Perhaps even more exciting, I was able to tell them something about our first attempts to measure the blood flow in these vessels without opening up the skull, a procedure that was for many years considered to be impossible. The new technique of transcranial Doppler sonography, which we were developing together with the Norwegian biocyberneticist, Dr. Rune Aaslid, was to prove to be one of the major advances in the struggle against cerebrovascular disease, offering new hope to the millions of stroke victims throughout the world. In the United States alone more than 170,000 people die each year as the result of a stroke, making it the third highest cause of death after heart disease and cancer. A further 200,000 are disabled and become a physical and spiritual burden to their relatives. Their care costs about $10 billion annually (87).

I looked at the slides with which I intended to end my lecture. Using the methodology of Doppler sonography, which was already widely applied by neurologists in continental Europe — but as yet little known in the United States — we were not only able to predict the risk of a stroke, but also the extent of what would happen to the patient as a result. Was I premature in showing cases where we were using this innovative technology, combined with the latest computer miracle, to produce a 3-dimensional image of the main blood vessels at the base of the human brain, which were colour-coded to show us where these life supporting arteries were becoming clogged?

I use the word "miracle" here in the sense that I use it for the take-off (or landing) of a Jumbo jet. Of course there are physical laws that can explain precisely why that gargantuan machine just does not drop out of the sky on landing at a speed so slow that it appears to be hovering in the air like a helicopter. But there is still something miraculous about this awe-inspiring sight. Since I had been closely involved with the development of the prototype Doppler ultrasound brain scanner, I was even more familiar with the physics involved in this. But each of those scans that we carried out on the first patients in 1984, represented to me nothing less than a minor miracle.

So these slides were the fireworks with which I was planning to end my introductory lecture. But, equally important, how should I start it? It was not easy to find a connection between the work that had taken over our lives for the past five years and the State of Texas. How far back did the physical laws go on which this methodology was based? Wasn't Doppler some sort of German scientist? When and where did he live? This could perhaps be a good opening narrative. The Americans have a great feel for history,

and who more than the Texans? So I reached for a medical dictionary that had served me well since my student days. It was a step that was to change my life more than I could have ever realised.

Under the entry for "Doppler" I read that the Doppler effect was named after "Christian Doppler, American mathematician, 1803—1853" (30). I was both surprised and elated at having found the ideal link between our modern technology from Europe being based on a 150 year-old mathematical observation of an American! But I was not convinced. So I reached for a further medical dictionary at hand for reassurance (82). This was only partially provided by the entry to the effect that "Christian J. Doppler, Austrian mathematician and physicist in America" was the gentleman in question. This rather took the shine off my planned opening remarks, but — even so — the basic work was obviously done here in America. So the next day I set out to learn more about this Austrian emigré. My search for Christian Doppler had begun.

It was a search that was to take me to four of the most beautiful cities in the world: Salzburg, Vienna, Prague and Venice. It was a search that was to give me entré to many doors through which the tourist or sightseer does not normally pass, to meet many people — unknown as well as famous — with whom I would have normally had no contact. It was a search that was to change the course, if only slightly, of my professional career. It was a search that led to the publication in 1988 of my first portrait of "Christian Doppler: Thinker and Benefactor" (36) which was to result in my being invited to all parts of the world to lecture on the unknown Austrian scientist whose name has become an established term in modern medical and other technologies.

The beginnings of this search, however, began in total confusion, which only increased as I consulted more literature references on the elusive Austrian. In attempting (unsuccessfully) to discover just where and when Doppler had been in America, I also found some confusion with his name. He was mostly referred to — as in the authoritative Encyclopedia Britannica — as Christian Johann Doppler, although many sources — including the equally authoritative Dictionary of Scientific Biography (90) — inverted the names to make him Johann Christian Doppler. Whilst most references gave his birth as being in Salzburg in 1803, some delayed this until 1805 (5, 89) or even 1808 (60). A further biographical dictionary (61) stated Doppler to be a "German physicist and mathematician", giving "Salzburg, Germany" as the place of birth and delaying the event by one day, as did the

Almanac of the Imperial Academy of Sciences in Vienna and others*. Greater consistency was shown with Venice being the place of death, although two authors (40, 89) did manage to transport this to Vienna, and several sources from Prague gave Doppler an extra year of life by giving 1854 as the year of death (11, 51, 84, 91), as does the official commemorative plaque on the site of his house there (page 36) and one author even extends it to 1858 (40). This last source also gives Doppler a period of tenure as Professor of Mathematics at Monaco!

My search, it seemed, could not be restricted to the narrow confines of a library. I suprised my wife by suddenly inviting her for a long weekend in Salzburg!

* *This was obviously based on details, probably from the year 1850, contained in Doppler's biographical file which are still in the Archives of the Austrian Academy of Sciences in Vienna. One of these is in Doppler's own handwriting and states: "I was born on 30th November 1803 in the City of Salzburg in the Crown State of Salzburg. Dr. Christian Doppler, Full Member of the Royal Academy." Karl Kreil was able to point out this surprising anomaly in his letter dated 12th April 1853 to Anton Schrötter, Secretary General of the Imperial Academy of Sciences (56) in time for him to give the correct birthdate in his obituary.*

From Toppler to Doppler: A Dynasty of Stonemasons

My first visit to Salzburg in search of Christian Doppler produced several surprises. Firstly, it was not easy to unearth traces of the — at least to me — famous scientist. Whilst many had heard of the name, and some knew that he was "some sort of physicist" or had even heard of the Doppler effect, I found none who knew more about the man or who were aware of the increasing significance of Doppler's work in medicine and other fields.

Certainly, the house in which he was born boasted a commemorative stone tablet, which was unveiled in 1903 in celebration of the 100th anniversary of that event (page 20). However, it is not known as "the Doppler House", but rather as "the Jetzelsberger House" after the family who had their business and lived in this historic building since the beginning of the century. It is to the present occupant, Frau Liselotte Jetzelsberger-Lanik, to whom we owe a great debt for her spirited efforts in preventing the demolition of the war-scarred house in 1946.

The square on which this house stands is not, as one would expect, called *Christian-Doppler-Platz*, but is named after a Salzburg painter, Hans Makart, whose life (1840—1884) postdates that of Doppler and who also has a nearby footbridge over the River Salzach named after hin, although his work is hardly known outside of Austria.

It is true that there is a *Christian-Doppler-Strasse* in Salzburg, but it is in a completely undistinguished area of that beautiful city which, due to its proximity to the gasworks, was heavily bombed in the Second World War, and gracelessy rebuilt at the end of hostilities. It is to be hoped that, in this jubilee year of Doppler's *magnum opus* which has, to paraphrase his own words, been of untold benefit to mankind, that a fitting memorial will be erected in the renamed *Christian-Doppler-Platz* on which the birthhouse stands. Certainly, Doppler's contribution has been considerably greater and farther reaching that that of Hans Makart, whose admirers should be content with the footbridge that bears his name. In the closing sentence of his foreword to the special edition of Doppler's work, published in Prague to celebrate the 100th anniversary of his birthday in 1903, Professor F. J. Studnička (85) pleaded: "Hopefully, a lasting monument will also be dedicated to him in the charming city of Mozart which rises from the banks of the torrential Salzach, proud of the merchant's son who first saw the light of day there 100 years ago." At the time of my first visit in 1985, however, neither the City Fathers nor the *Bürger* of Salzburg were aware that their

city had begotten within its walls a man whose scientific achievement can make claim to equal the musical genius of its other famous son, Wolfgang Amadeus Mozart.

The second surprise was to discover that, although traces of the scientist Christian Doppler were scanty in the Salzburg area, there was no scarcity of records of the other members of his family who were — almost without exception — stonemasons. The patriach of this dynasty was Andreas (Andrä) Doppler who has been mistakenly reported by several authors (including this one!) to have come to the Salzburg area from Bavaria in 1674. It is from the hobby genealogist, Bartholomäus Reischel of Wals (72), that we learn of the first records of Andreas Doppler being those of his marriage in 1670 in Viehhausen, near Salzburg, where he had just opened his stonemason's workshop. Like his wife, Maria, Andreas Doppler had come to the hamlet of Viehhausen from Grossgmain on the Austrian-Bavarian border, where his father, Adam Toppler, had been a farmer since 1635, when he had inherited the farm from his brother Wolf. Wolf and his wife Barbara had died of the plague, as apparently did his father Leonhart Toppler, together with his wife and all other children of the family. This farmer Leonhart Toppler provides the earliest records, dated 1605, that we have of the family. It was with the moving of his great nephew Andrä from Grossgmain to Viehhausen, that from the farming Topplers the dynasty of the Doppler stonemasons was to grow.

Following the birth of their second daughter in 1675, Andreas and Maria Doppler moved to the house and stonemason's workshop that he had built in the newly-named settlement of Himmelreich in the parish of Wals, which is where the airport of Salzburg is now located. It was here, two years later, that their son Georg — the great grandfather of Christian Doppler — was born.

For the visitor with time and interest enough to look around Himmelreich and the neighbouring villages, there are several surviving works of the Doppler stonemasons in this area. The oldest are in the town of Grossgmain, near the Bavarian border, where the Topplers tilled their farm. Here, on the pavement outside the village church, stands an unusual baroque fountain with a double figure of a Madonna carved by Johann Schwaiger of Reichenhall. The decorative fruit and cherubs' heads on the bowl and pedestal are the work of Andreas Doppler from the year 1693 (54). It was only after I reported this fact in my earlier portrait of Christian Doppler (36), that I became aware that in the church itself are examples of the work of three generations of Dopplers going back to 1675 (8). In this year Andreas Doppler made a frame for the sacristy door in pale marble.

His son Georg has many examples of his handiwork in this church, including the choir altar behind the high altar (1711) and the right side altar (1734). He also laid the red and yellow marble floor in 1748. His son Joseph (born September 2, 1732) made two marble offertory boxes for the church in 1794.

Joseph Doppler took over the stonemasonry from his father in 1754 and extended the house in 1762 to accommodate the guests in the inn *(Gasthof Himmelreich)* for which he received the licence in that year. His magnificent marble altar can be seen in the Sacellum chapel of the university building in the *Hofstallgasse* opposite the Festival Theatre *(Festspielhaus)*. It was carried out in 1768 for the Prince Archbishop of Salzburg, Sigismund von Schrattenbach, from a design of Wolfgang Hagenauer (83).

In 1796 (48) among the possessions of Joseph Doppler were catalogued: "Doppler, Stonemason in the so-called Himmelreich, possesses by the Untersberg, on the meadows of Wals and close to the road to Reichenhall and Tyrol, two marble quarries, in one of which is a red and white flecked and also a multicoloured marble and in the other a white marble is quarried. For this he pays a lease to the Court of the High Prince of 13 Kreutzer for each foot of white marble and 6 Kreutzer for the multicoloured. From this stone he himself makes altars, portals, tombstones, window frames and the like."

Marble is still quarried at the foot of the *Untersberg* which we approach by the *Dopplerstrasse*, finally arriving by the steep *Dopplersteig* (Doppler's Climb) and there is still a stonemason's yard in Himmelreich, now in the possession of the Gollackner family into whose hands it passed by marriage in 1836 (72). Until recently there was still a *Gasthaus Himmelreich* opposite, where the Doppler's inn had stood, but it was part of the modern Hotel Himmelreich, which has itself now been demolished to make way for the development of an "Airport Centre". Since street names were introduced in Himmelreich in 1974, there has been an *Andrä-Doppler-Weg*.

In the hamlet of Viehhausen, where Andreas Doppler first set up in the stonemason's trade, there is a small chapel dedicated to the Holy Trinity with a beautiful marble altar bearing the inscription: "To the Glory of the Most Holy Trinity and to Mary, Mother of God, Georg Dopler*, Master

* *The spelling of the name with only one letter "p" is apparently without significance, since there was considerable variation in the spelling of names in those times. We have seen how the name Toppler evolved into Doppler, and in the records of the birth of Georg Doppler (5th May 1677) the father is noted as "Andreas Dobler, Stonemason in Himmelreich". The name is also stated as "Dopler" in the records of Christian Doppler's birth and baptism (page 22).*

Stonemason in Himmelreich, has Erected this Altar". This chapel, which was originally built in 1625 by a Salzburg trader as thanks for being spared by the plague, was destroyed in 1663 by an oak which was felled in a storm. Rebuilt by another Salzburg tradesman, it was then burnt down after being struck by lightning in 1710, to be erected in its present form in 1714, at which time Andrä Doppler's son Georg donated the altar.

In this chapel on 26th November 1792, by special permission of the consistory, Johann Evangelist Doppler, master stonemason of Salzburg, married Theresia Seeleuthner before his grandfather's altar. The witnesses were the groom's father, Joseph, and Theresia's employer, Franz Gschwendtner, who was a member of the Salzburg City Council. As a result of this union, eleven years later, their third child and second son was born at 11 o'clock in the morning of 29th November 1803. He was predestined to become the first scientist in this dynasty of stonemasons.

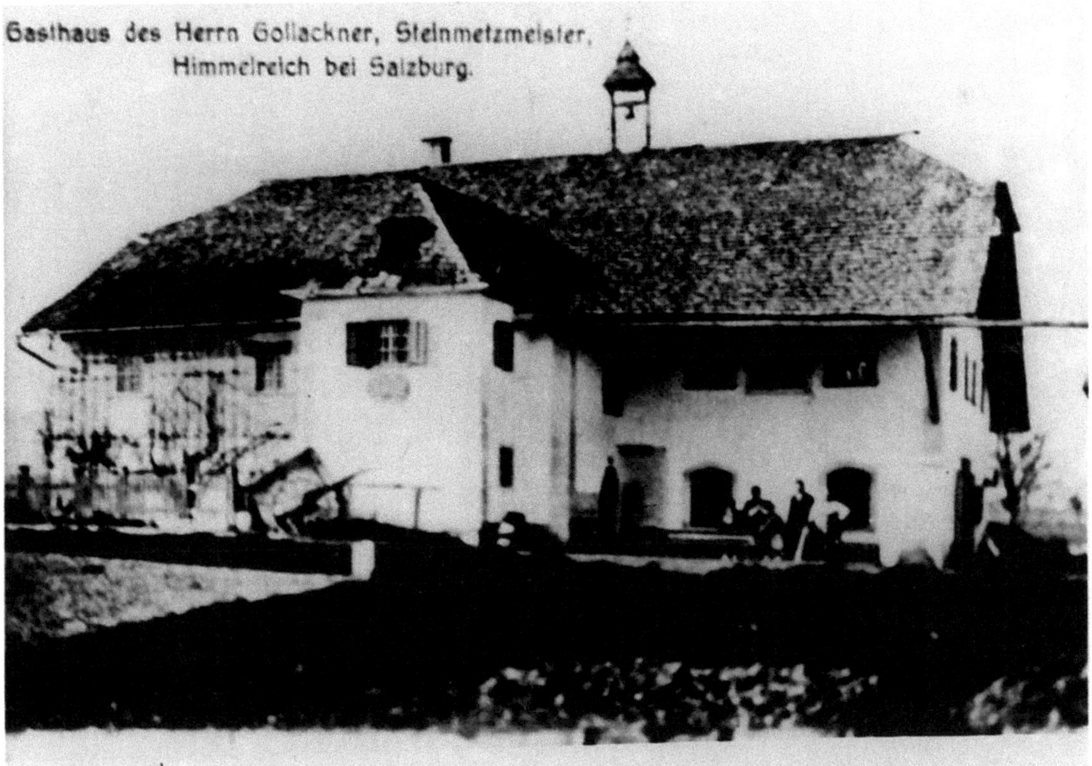

The house in Himmelreich near Salzburg inhabited by Christian Doppler's ancestors from 1675 until 1792 when the Doppler House in Salzburg was completed in its present form (see plans on pages 18—19). The part of the building on the right housed the stonemasonry and the guesthouse occupied the middle part.

(Reproduced from a postcard kindly provided by the late Ludwig Gollackner, Master Stonemason of Himmelreich near Salzburg)

Salzburg: The Young Doppler

In 1788 Joseph Doppler took possession of the single-storey building set into the city wall of Salzburg which had previously been the "Hut of the official Court Stonemason". This had been sold off, together with other buildings and the Court Marble Quarries at the *Untersberg*, as an economy measure by the Prince Archbishop Schrattenbach and was previously in the hands of another stone craftsman, Jakob Mösl. He had wanted to add a further floor to the building, but was unsuccessful in his attempts (both in 1761 and again in 1767) to obtain permission due to the opposition of the house owners on either side. It appears that planning permission was a source of neighbourly animosity even in those days!

Jakob Mösl died in 1787 and the house was inherited by his widow and children from whom Joseph Doppler obtained it the following year (53). He, too, wanted to extend the building, but met with the same opposition from the neighbours as did his predecessor when he applied for permission to add three further floors. A less ambitious application for only two additional floors (pages 18—19) was approved by the authorities in 1791 and completed within a few months. It is not known if this was supervised by Joseph Doppler or his son Johann Evangelist, also a master stonemason. In any event, it was Johann who took possession of the completed house in 1792, leaving the running of the family business in Himmelreich to his elder brother Mathias and his wife Theresia when their father died in January of 1798. These were to be the last members of the Doppler stonemason dynasty in Himmelreich. Due to mounting debts the stonemasonry, together with other property of the Dopplers, fell into the hands of their creditors who sold it in September 1803 to the master stonemason Mathias Waldhütter and his wife Elisabeth (72).

This house still stands in fine condition on what is now the Makart Platz, but it was the Hannibal Platz when the Dopplers lived there. Although the house has not changed significantly since it was built (page 21), the surroundings certainly have. The Dopplers were able to look out across the River Salzach to an unbroken and breathtaking view of the old city — a view that was completely blocked by the building of the hotel *Österreichischer Hof* in 1866. The view in the other direction, however, has since been considerably improved by the demolition of the city loan office in 1906 to reveal the Church of the Holy Trinity in its full stateliness. The house in which the Mozart family lived on the southeast side of the square was badly damaged by a bombing raid in the Second World War and partly

rebuilt in an ugly fashion. Plans to restore it to its original state are now well advanced.

At 3 o'clock in the afternoon of 29th November 1803, Johann Evangelist Doppler, who was then 37 years old, took his third child and second son, who had been born at 11 o'clock that morning in the house of the prosperous stonemason in the *Hannibal Platz*, to the Church of St. Andrä, barely a two-minute walk along the *Dreifaltigkeitsgasse*, through the Sauter Archway to the junction with the *Linzer Gasse* where the church stood. Accompanied by his chosen Godmother, the trader Anna Zezi, Johann Doppler asked the chaplain Georg Lang to baptise the baby with the names Christian Andreas.

The old Church of St. Andrä no longer stands. It was pulled down in 1862 in order to widen the streets of that increasingly busy part of old Salzburg. We are told that the font in which Doppler was baptised was taken to the new Church of St. Andrä (81) when this was consecrated in 1898. It was here in this graceless building on the Mirabellplatz, rendered even more ugly by bomb damage in 1944—1945, that I found the records of births and baptisms at the beginning of my search for Christian Doppler in the Spring of 1985.

These refuted beyond all doubt the names "Christian Johann" or even "Johann Christian" that had been used in the majority of biographical and other documentation on Doppler (44, 70, 77, 89), as does the fact that Christian's elder brother, born nine years previously, had already been given the name Johann after his father. The earliest use of this misnomer that I have been able to find is in an astronomical journal published in Berlin in 1896 (74) and it has been perpetuated by many eminent scientists and historians of whom one would expect greater care in checking basic facts. It has been suggested (45) that the mistake originated by careless reading of the entry in the records of St. Andrä (page 22) whereby the dividing vertical lines of the columns in this book were overlooked and the first name of the father (Johann) was misread as the second name of the son. It seems that my reporting of the correct name in a letter to a medico-scientific journal in 1985 (33) was the first time that this has appeared in print.

There are a number of reasons that Johann and Therese Doppler might have chosen to name their second son Andreas. It was probably in continuance of the family tradition — practised in all previous generations — of naming a son after the patriach of the dynasty of stonemasons who first

entered that craft in 1670. Or it could have been to honour the Holy St. Andreas, patron saint of the church in which he was baptised and whose saint's day was celebrated on the following day. However, in the numerous records I have examined it has not been possible to find one single example of Doppler ever using his second name — even in such formal documents as the family registration form in Prague (page 49) and the records of his marriage. He usually signed himself simply as "Doppler" or sometimes "Christian Doppler".

What were young Christian Doppler's earliest recollections of his home in Salzburg, where he grew up with his elder brother Johann and two older sisters, Katharina and Theresia, the fifth child Anna following almost five years after Doppler's birth? They must have been those of the noise and bustle of the stonemason's trade that was carried out on the ground floor of the house (see plans on page 18) and of the almost continuous building that was required to make extensions to the workshops and other rooms which were necessary to accommodate the flourishing business (14). Father Doppler had already received the Prize of the Viennese Academy of Art in 1782 (86) and was working on many important commissions, as well as supplying marble from the *Untersberg* for the magnificent palaces and court buildings of King Ludwig of Bavaria (14).

A further stonemason's workshop was later opened in the *Griesgasse* on the other side of the River Salzach, less than five minutes walk from the Doppler home. It can be easily identified by its beautifully crafted marble portal on this street (it is now number 8) and if one passes through into the courtyard, also decorated with small remnants of the stonemason's craft, one comes across the old workshop with a less ornate marble portal with an inscription informing us that this was: "The Stonemason's Workshop of Joh: Doppler." This does not refer to Christian Doppler's father or older brother, but to his nephew who took over the lease of the workshop in 1858 on the death of the master stonemason Anton Högler, who had been appointed the official guardian of Christian Doppler when his father died in 1823.

It apparently became a tradition in the Salzburg branch of the stonemason's dynasty that the eldest son, who was intended to lead the family business, was baptised "Johann Evangelist", after Christian Doppler's father and brother who founded it. The last two stonemasons of this name and lineage (who died in 1892 and 1928 respectively) share a family grave in the Communial Cemetery in Salzburg, together with a Doppler daughter, Johanna, who died as recently as 1942.

It is, however, in the beautiful cemetery of St. Sebastian, not far from the Doppler home, where Mozart's father and wife are buried — as well as the medieval medical researcher Philipp Theophrast Bombast von Hohenheim, better known as Paracelsus — that the most immediate members of Doppler's family are to be found. His father, who died in the house on the Hannibal Platz in January 1823, when Christian was 19 and studying at the Polytechnic in Vienna, is buried here, but the gravestone can no longer be located. The grave of his brother who died in 1838 at the age of 44 is still clearly legible in the colonnades, and from it we see that it is shared by his widow Anna, who was to outlive him by 25 years, and six of their ten children who died in infancy. Further along these colonnades, Christian's elder sister Katharina (died 1873, aged 76) and his younger sister Anna (died 1886, aged 78) share their resting places with their husbands, each of whom predeceased them by one year.

In the graveyard around them are many examples of the Dopplers' handiwork, with their names inscribed in various forms on the gravestones they made. Most commonly it is simply "Doppler", sometimes "J. Doppler" or "Joh: Doppler", and one can ascertain from the dates engraved to which particular head of the family business they refer. One of them, dated 1843, bears the name "Anna Doppler" at the foot, indicating that Doppler's sister-in-law ran the business following her husband's early death, until their eldest son Johann was experienced enough to take it over. It was in this busy world of stonemasonry that Christian Doppler spent his youthful years, and it was originally intended that he should also learn the stonemason's craft (14). His grandson, Dr. Adolf Doppler, tells us that he would spend hours at the churchyard, sketching the angels that he would later model in clay at the stonemason's yard. One is tempted to ask if living and growing up in the dusty enviroment of the stonemason's trade did not perhaps sow the seed of the pulmonary disease from which he was to die at the age of 49? The fact that in the entry of his father's death in the records of the Church of St. Andrä in Salzburg we can read that the cause of death was "lung disease", as was the death of his brother Johann in 1838, would seem to confirm that Doppler succumbed to this notorious occupational hazard of stonemasons.

It was already apparent before his teens that Christian Doppler's frail physique and recurrent ill health did not fit him for the robust physical work that stonemasonry involves. At the age of 13, with his elementary education completed, Doppler's father decided that his second son was not suitable to follow in his trade and sent him for three years (1816—1819) to the "German School" in Salzburg. Here he received a medallion for out-

standing scholastic ability and in 1820 he attended the 4th grade of a secondary school in Linz. From grandson Adolf Doppler (13) we also have the information that he then spent two years (1821—1822) as a commercial apprentice, but confirmation of this cannot be found elsewhere*. It seems that his father wanted his son to look after the business side of the family stonemasonry. It was probably at about this time that Johann Doppler consulted Simon Stampfer, who was teaching mathematics at the Lyceum in Salzburg, to test the young Christian's aptitude for such a career.

This was to prove an important milestone in Doppler's life, for Stampfer recognised the lad's capabilities in mathematics and his suitability for a scientific education. As a result of Stamper's enthusiastic advice, Christian Doppler was sent to the Polytechnic Institute in Vienna in 1822, just a few months before his 19th birthday. Here he attended lectures on mathematics, mechanics and physics. From the reports of the Polytechnic we learn that Doppler was extremely industrious and obtained the highest grades. One of these reports reads: "His extraordinarily hard work and excellent moral behaviour single him out for special commendation."

Doppler himself, however, was not so enthusiastic about what he was later to call "a one-sided education" which failed to provide him with the intellectual stimulus he was seeking. After two and a quarter years in Vienna he returned to his native Salzburg in January 1825. Here, at the age of 21, he decided to complete his formal education at a private high school.

Because of his age and maturity, as well as the excellent grades he had obtained at the Polytechnic, he was given special permission to sit the examinations considerably sooner than the six years laid down in the regulations, and he successfully completed the course in half of that time. The following obligatory course in philosophical studies he completed in two years (80). During this latter period he supported himself by giving lessons in mathematics and physics at St. Rupert's College. At the same time he was learning modern languages — French, Italian and English — as well as commerce and accounting with a local trader!

Also during this time Doppler began to write poetry and essays, which he possibly submitted to local journals and newspapers for publication. Some of these were copied and saved by his grandson Adolf. They vary from

* *It should be pointed out here that Dr. Adolf Doppler is not always a completely reliable source of information. He tended to exaggerate the achievements of his grandfather and, for example, gives an incorrect date for his marriage (page 39).*

"Lines composed on the wedding festivities of my brother Johann Doppler to Anna Maria Freundelsperger on 16th January 1826", to sensitive poems composed on the death of friends and colleagues (each commencing: "Why are you weeping? He still lives!") and a pair of poems entitled "Satisfaction" and "Dissatisfaction". A handwritten manuscript of an essay from about this time, entitled: "An Attempt at a Geographic-Technological Painting" has recently come into the possession of the Christian Doppler Foundation in Salzburg.

Another essay is of special interest: "On a strange characteristic of the human eye", which Doppler's grandson dates as being written between 1825 and 1828, when Doppler was in his early twenties. He comments: "This work contains the independent discovery of the 'blind spot' of the eye by Christian Doppler. He himself says in this essay that he can hardly believe that this fact has not yet been discovered, and says of this phenomenon 'that it must be almost the only one to which man is led through its own nature'. He never published this work. Perhaps he became aware that this phenomenon was discovered at about the middle of the 17th century by von Mariotte. In any case, this work can claim to be of historical value. It represents a youthful work of Christian Doppler."

On completion of his philosophical studies in 1829 he went off again to Vienna — already in his mid-twenties — to begin his assistantship at the Polytechnic Institute there.

The original plans (1791) of Christian Doppler's birth-house which was completed the following year. It was built within the city walls of Salzburg.

The heading reads:

PLAN and ELEVATION
of the previous Court — since then Mösl — and now Doppler Stone-mason's Hut and Quarters on the city wall by the Lederer Gateway, following the proposed building of new living accommodation.

(From the Salzburg State Archives)

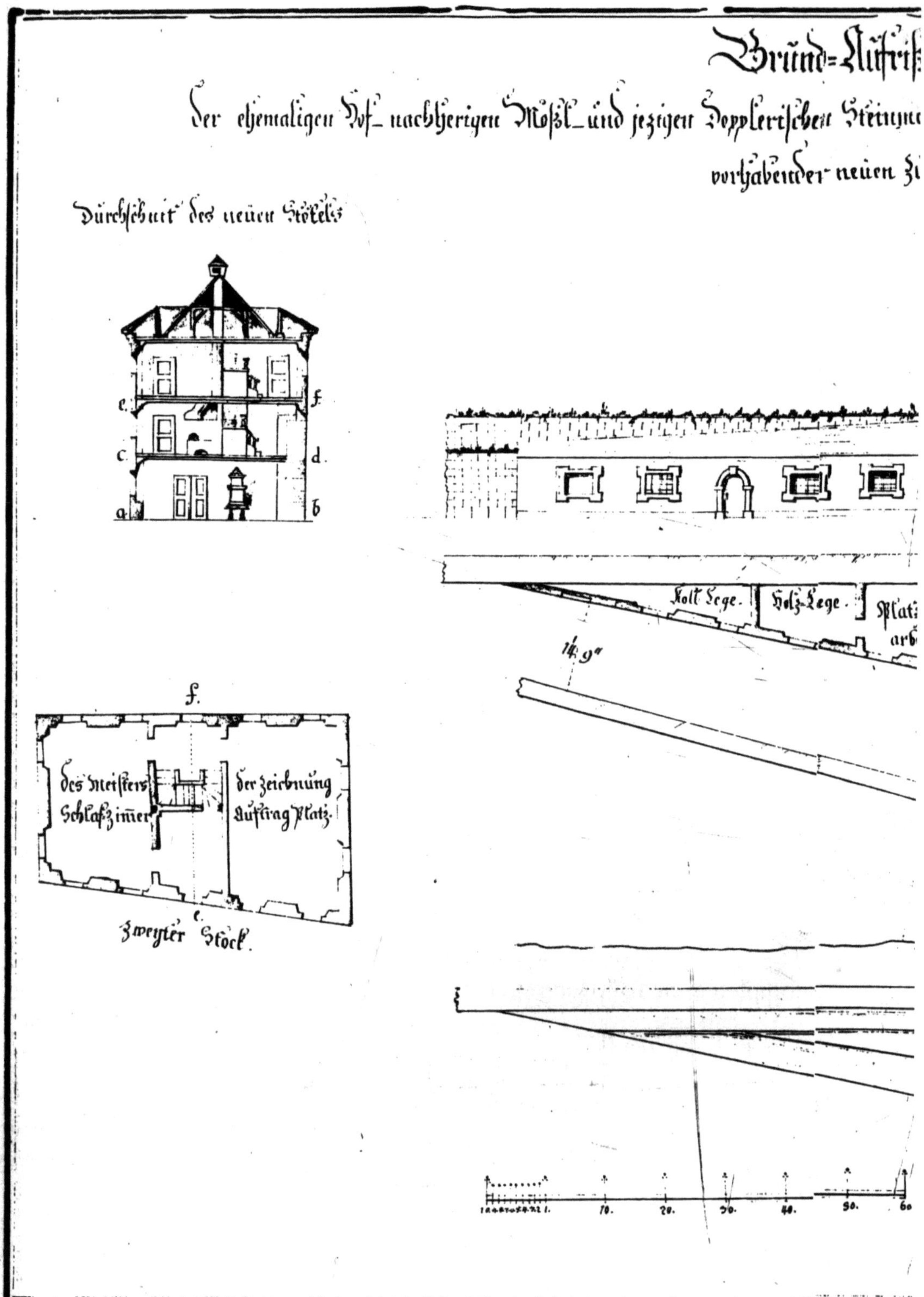
Grund-Aufriß
der ehemaligen Hof- nachherigen Mößl- und jezigen Dopplerischen Steinme
vorhabender neuen Zi
Durchschnitt des neuen Stöckels
Kohl-Lege.
Holz-Lege.
Platz
arb
14. 9"
des Meisters Schlafzimer
der Zeichnung Auftrag Platz.
Zweyter Stock.
10. 20. 30. 40. 50. 60

Durchschnitt

…itte und Wohnung, an der Stadtmauer neben dem Leederer-Thore, nach

…ung des Stöckels ~.

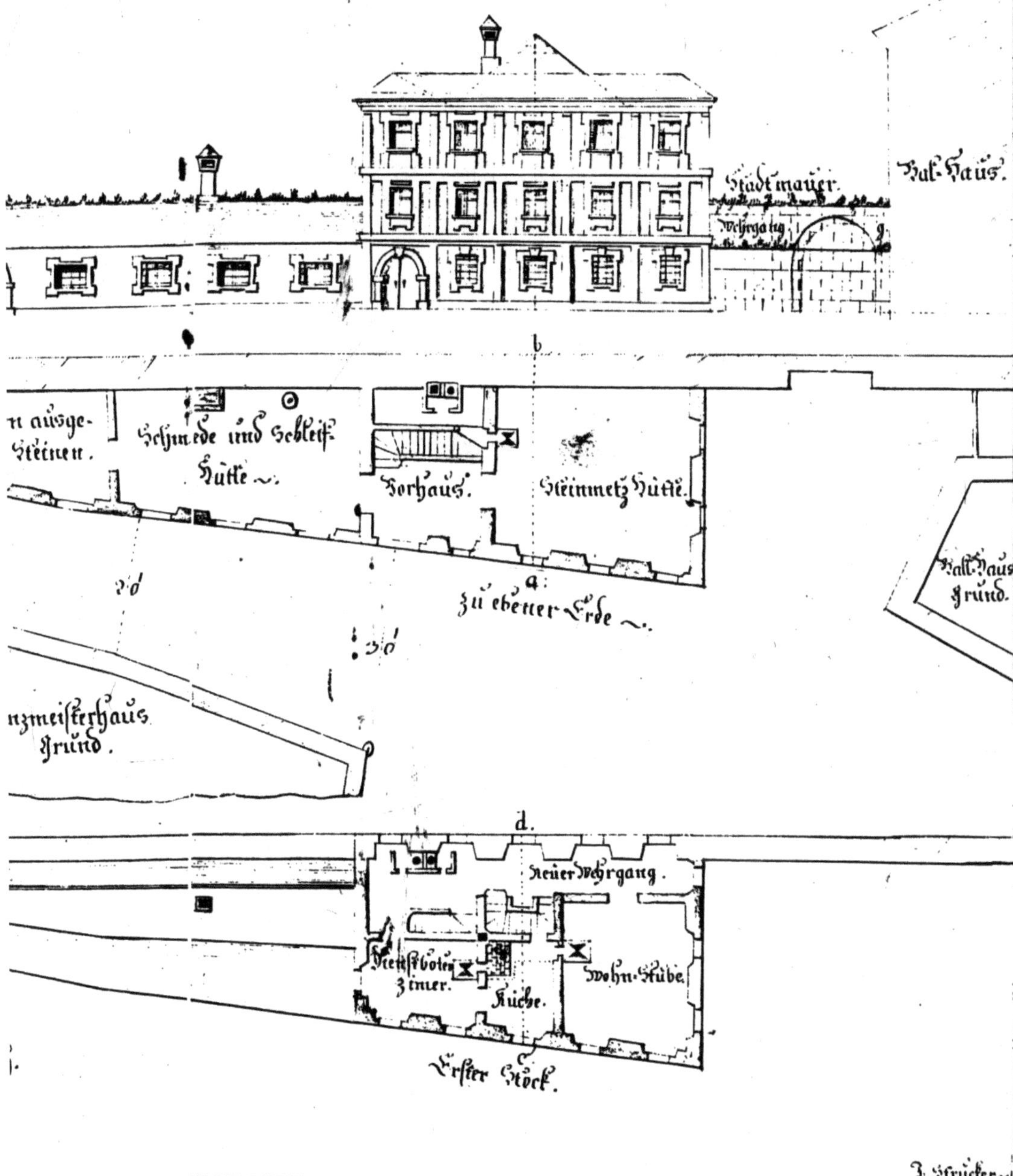

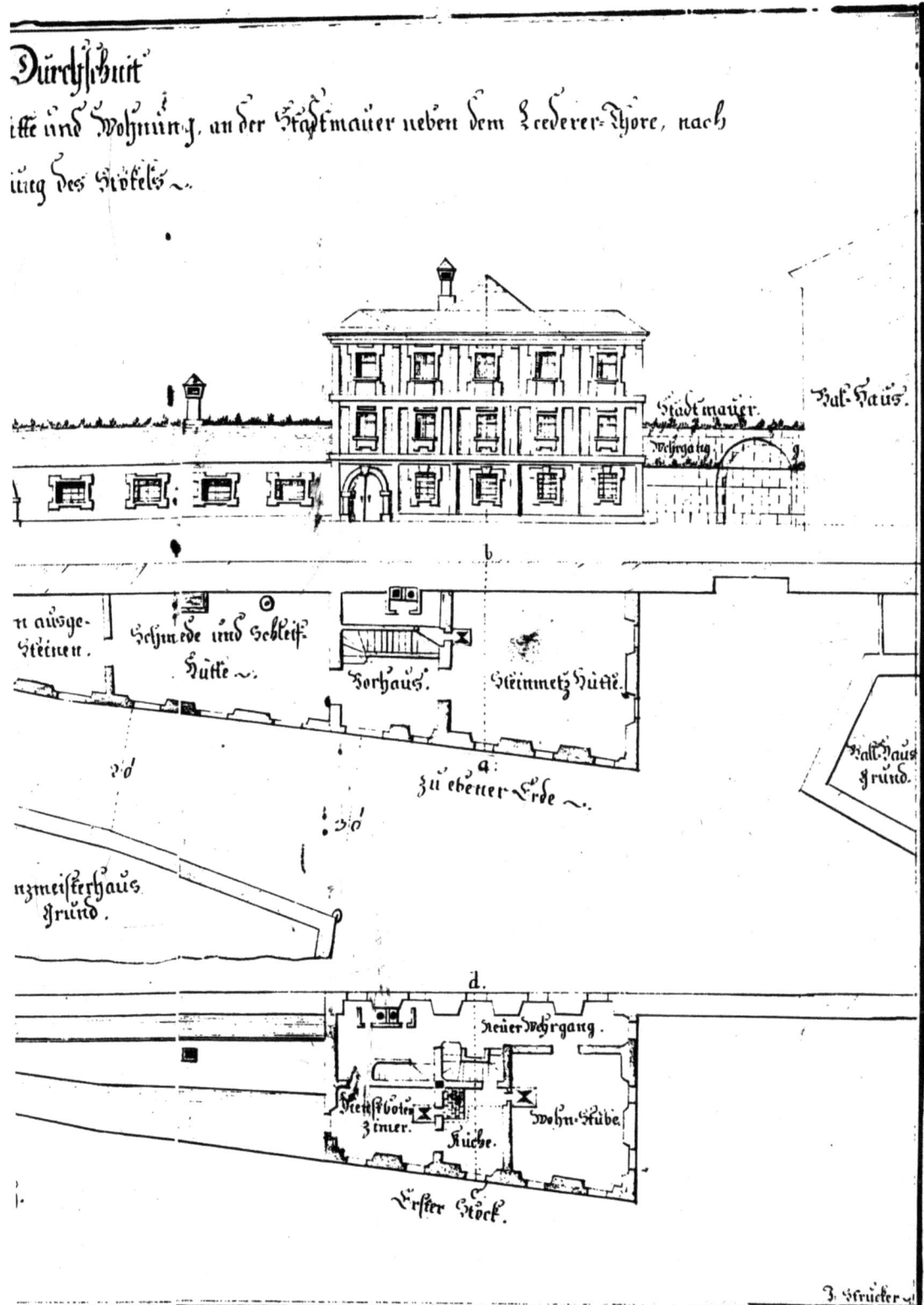

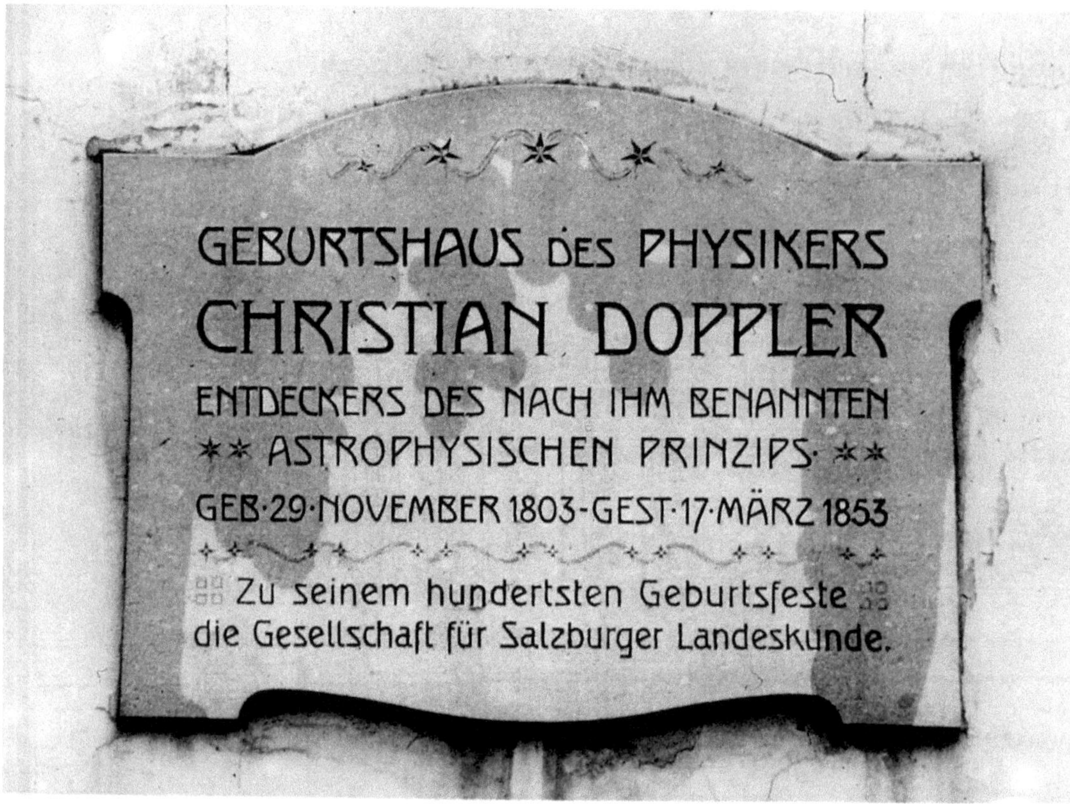
GEBURTSHAUS DES PHYSIKERS
CHRISTIAN DOPPLER
ENTDECKERS DES NACH IHM BENANNTEN
** ASTROPHYSISCHEN PRINZIPS **
GEB·29·NOVEMBER 1803-GEST·17·MÄRZ 1853
Zu seinem hundertsten Geburtsfeste
die Gesellschaft für Salzburger Landeskunde.

The commemorative tablet mounted on the side of the Doppler House in 1903 in celebration of the 100th anniversary of Christian Doppler's birth. It reads:

BIRTH-HOUSE of the PHYSICIST
CHRISTIAN DOPPLER
DISCOVERER OF THE ASTROPHYSICAL
PRINCIPLE NAMED AFTER HIM
Born: 29th NOVEMBER 1803 — Died: 17th MARCH 1853

(Photograph by the author)

The Doppler House as it stands today on the Makart Platz in Salzburg — not significantly changed from the original design of 1791 (above).

(Photograph by the author)

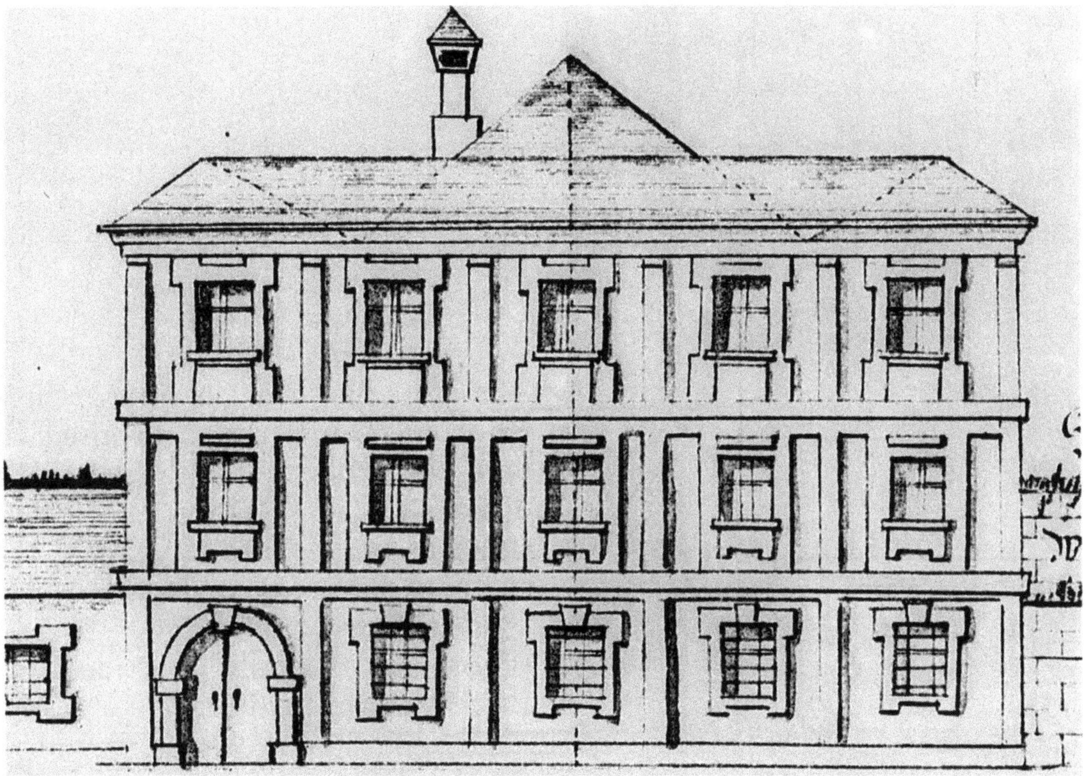

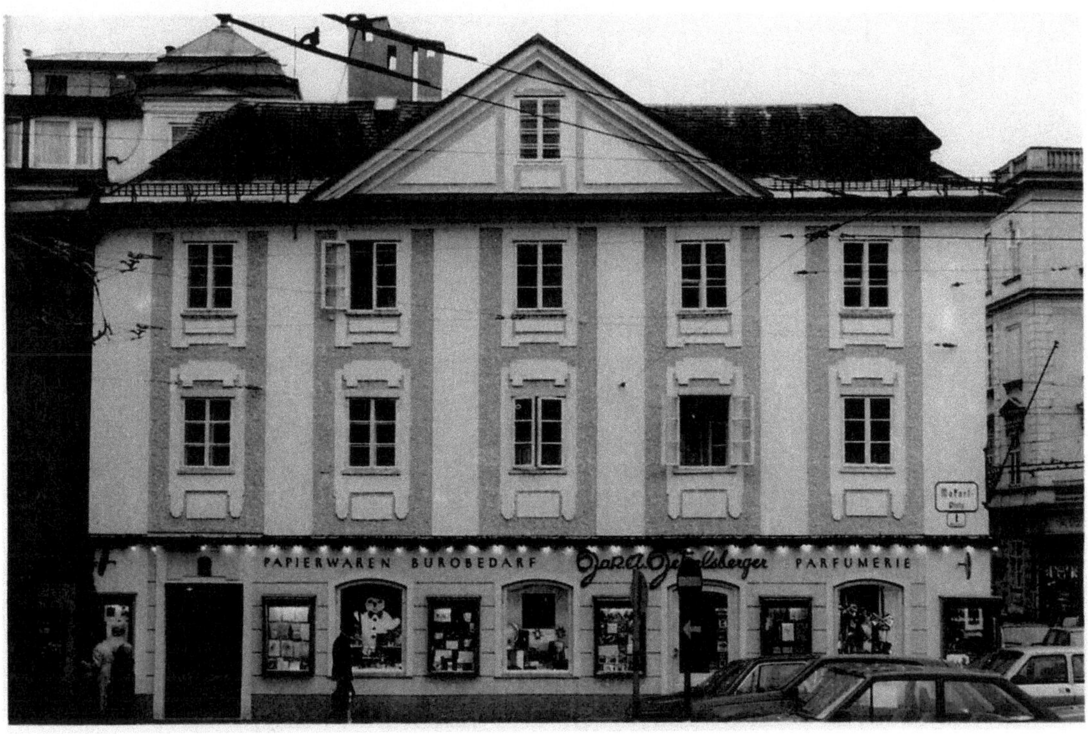
PAPIERWAREN BUROBEDARF
PARFUMERIE

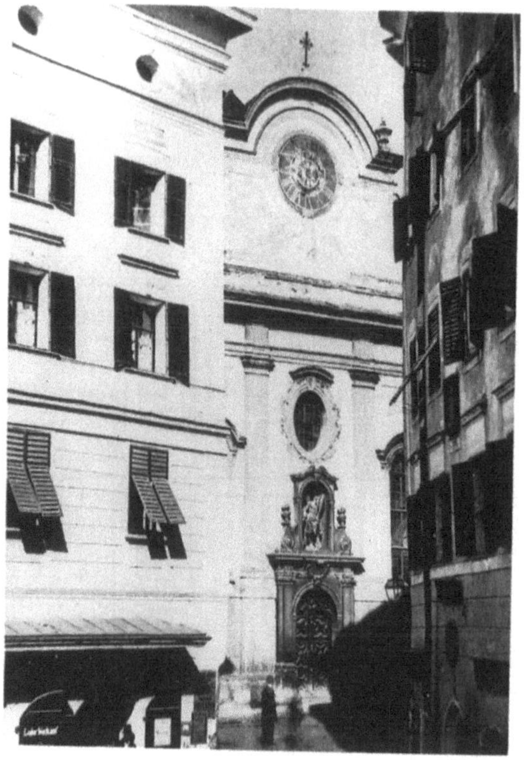

The old Church of St. Andrä where Christian Doppler was baptised. It (and the building on the left) was demolished in 1862 to enable the street to be widened. It is now the site of a shoe shop.

(Photograph kindly provided by Peter Matern, Salzburg)

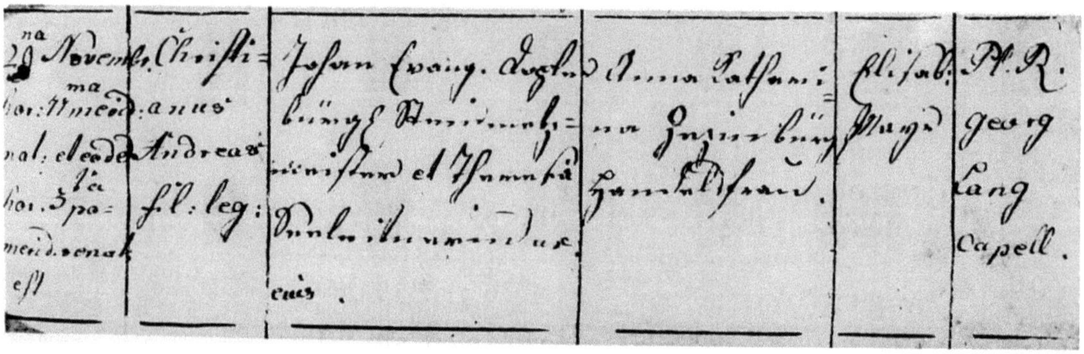

29na Novembr. | Christianus Andreas fil. leg: | Georg Lang Capell.

The original entry of the birth and baptism of Christian Andreas Doppler on 29th November 1803.

(From the records of the Church of St. Andrä, Salzburg)

Eb. Stadtpfarramt Salzburg-St. Andrä
Telefon Nr. 71375 — Postsparkassenkonto Nr. 6996

ZAHL: ....   SALZBURG, am ....

Auszug aus dem Taufuch St. Andrä, Salzburg, Band V. Seite 29

Christian Andreas D o p l e r ,
geboren am 29. 11. 1803 11 Uhr vormittag,
getauft am selben Tag um 3 Uhr nachmittag.

Eltern: Johann Evangelist Dopler, XXX bürgerlicher Steinmetz-
meister und Therese Seeleitner, dessen Ehefrau.

Patin : Anna Katharina Zezi, bürgerliche H‸ndelsfrau,
Hebamme : Elisabeth Mayr,
Taufender Priester: Pf.R. Georg Lang, Capell.

A modern extract from the records of baptism in the Church of St. Andrä. It reads:

> Christian Andreas Dopler
> born on 29. 11. 1803 at 11 a. m.
> baptised on the same day at 3 p. m.
>
> Parents: Johann Evangelist Dopler, master
> stonemason and Therese Seeleitner, his wife.
>
> Godmother: Anna Katherina Zezi, trader,
> Midwife: Elisabeth Mayr
> Baptising priest: Rev. R. Georg Lang, Chaplain.

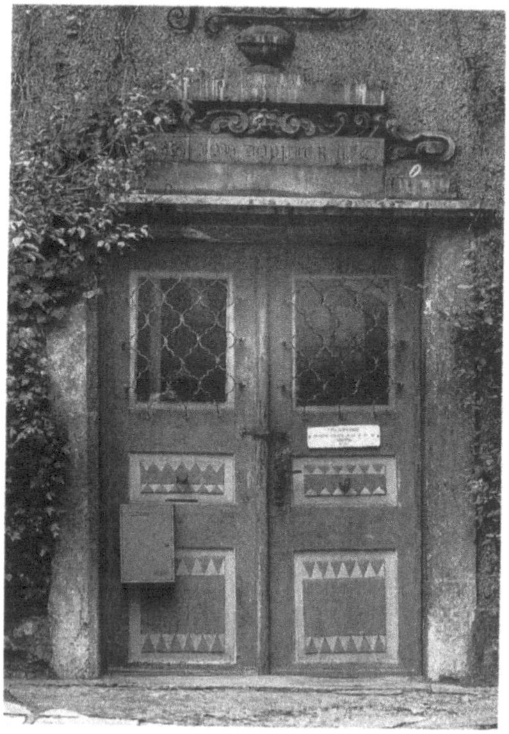

The building in the yard of *Griesgasse 8* in Salzburg. The inscription above the doorway (lower picture) reads:
The Stonemason's Workshop of
Joh: Doppler

(Photograph by Carla Endl, Salzburg)

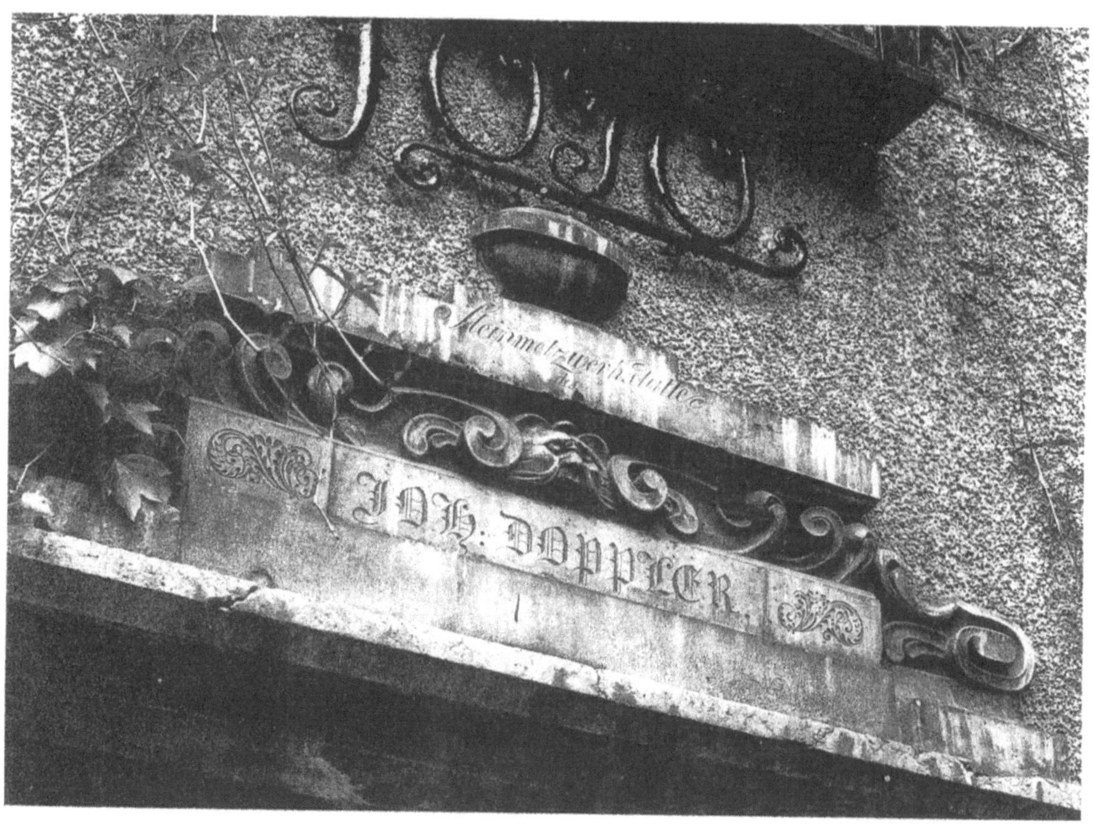

Vienna: Hope and Disappointment

Already in 1825, following his studies at the Polytechnic Institute in Vienna, Doppler had applied for an assistantship in pure higher mathematics there with Professor Joseph Hantschl. We know from his report on the four candidates, dated 20th October 1825, which is in the archives of the Technical University, that while he spoke highly of Doppler's mathematical achievements, he pointed out that since he had spent almost a year in Salzburg "Devoted to his Latin studies", he would have had very little time for mathematical work during that time. This absence also meant that Hantschl had no opportunity to judge his abilities to lecture. The post was given to another candidate, Karl Lamla, and in November Doppler received his first letter of rejection, but which was by no means to be the last.

On June 14, 1829, Doppler applied once again from Salzburg for an assistantship at the Polytechnic Institute, this time with Professor Adam von Burg, who had until the previous year taught him at the Salzburg Lyceum. In August von Burg expressed his preference for Doppler over the other candidate, and in September he took up his first position with the usual annual salary of 400 Guilders plus 60 Guilders accommodation allowance, for an initial period of two years. In November of that year he also received permission to give paid tuition in elementary mathematics to students at the Polytechnic.

In July 1831 this two-year period came to an end and Doppler applied for and received an extension for a further two years. It was during this time that Doppler published his first scientific works, the first being "A Contribution to the Theory of Parallels" which appeared in the Yearbook of the Vienna Polytechnic in 1832 (15) together with two other purely mathematical contributions. The following year his paper on "The Probable Cause of Excitation of Electricity through Contact" was also published in the Yearbook (16).

Already early in 1833, approaching the age of 30, Doppler started applying for teaching positions which he could take over when he left the Polytechnic in September. The first of these was the position of Professor of Mathematics and Nautical Theory which became vacant in February of that year at the Imperial Nautical Academy in Trieste, with the interviews and examinations being held at the Polytechnic Institute in Vienna. Doppler took part in these, but in July received notice of his rejection.

When he left Vienna in October he had not yet been successful in obtaining a position, and the year 1834 marked the lowest point in Doppler's career. Despite numerous applications, he was still unsuccessful in finding a teaching appointment and was compelled to work as a bookkeeper at the cotton-spinning factory of Wachtl & Co. near Bruck on the River Leitha. At the end of the year he had given up all hope of finding a suitable position in Europe and accompanied his brother Johann on a visit to Munich, where he discussed with the American Consul the possibilities of finding a job in the New World.

He had already sold most of his possessions — including his books — to finance his journey, when news reached him of two appointments that were offered: one was as Professor of Higher Mathamatics and Physics at the Secondary School in Bern, and the other as Professor of Elementary Mathematics and Commercial Accounting at the State Secondary School in Prague. We are told that, although the post in Switzerland commanded a higher salary, it was out of a sense of patriotism that Doppler accepted the position in Prague, which was then part of the Austrian Empire (58), to which he received the official appointment on 9th February 1835. Doppler was one of 14 applicants for this post and passed the examinations in all subjects with the grade "excellent". He was particularly brilliant in the mathematical questions, and his lecture was graded as "good and comprehensible".

Doppler gave up all ideas of going to America and never left the Austrian Empire.

Prague and the Coloured Light of the Double Stars

On 30th April 1835 Christian Doppler took his oath as a teacher of elementary mathematics and commercial accounting at the State Secondary School in Prague. The starting annual salary of 800 Guilders, which in the following January rose to 1,000 Guilders, obviously made it possible for him to marry in that year Mathilde Sturm, the daughter of a Salzburg gold and silversmith, and the first of their five children, also Mathilde, was born on 22nd January 1837 (see next chapter, "The Doppler Family").

Early in the same year Doppler was appointed to the position of Supplementary Professor of Higher Mathematics and Practical Geometry at the Prague Technical Institute and published three works in Baumgartner's Journal of Physics. But this picture of apparent family bliss and professional advancement is somewhat deceptive, and we read that Doppler was not at all happy in Prague (84), having to carry a very large burden of teaching duties of eight weekly lectures for about 400 students and to examine them all individually without assistance. The astronomer Karl Kreil, who was in Prague throughout this time, mentioned in a letter written shortly after Doppler's death (27th April 1853) to the Secretary General of the Imperial Academy of Sciences in Vienna, Anton Schrötter (56): "His ill health began already in Prague, where numerous lectures before a large number of listeners, in small overcrowded rooms, began to take toll of his health." Professor Schrötter included this in his obituary presented at a special commemorative meeting of the Imperial Academy of Sciences held on 30th May, and added: "The seed of the illness which led to his early death grew in him here." This may be true, but — as this author has already commented (33) — the seed was certainly sown during Doppler's youthful years in the stonemason's house in Salzburg.

Early in 1836 the restless Doppler had already begun to apply for professorships in mathematics at Laibach, Görz and other cities (42) and in May 1837 he took part in an interview and examination for the post of Professor of Higher Mathematics, as the successor to Adam von Burg at the Polytechnic Institute in Vienna, but in August Josef Salomon was appointed to this post. Between April 1836 and August 1837 Doppler made three further unsuccessful applications and Dr. Adolf Doppler complained that his grandfather was at a disadvantage due to his lack of nerves in this stressful atmosphere of competitiveness.

On 25th September 1837 the mathematician and philosopher Bernard Bolzano wrote to the Secretary of the Royal Bohemian Society of Sciences, recommending the publication of one of Doppler's mathematical works in the proceedings of the Society and recommending him for full membership (4). This letter, however, apparently did not comply with the rules of the Society as a formal proposal for membership and it was not until 28th June 1840 that twelve full members met to vote on the full and associate membership of a number of applicants, including Karl Kreil and Christian Doppler. Following a number of unanimous or large majority votes (Kreil received eleven votes with one against), Doppler and three other candidates were elected with the worst result of seven votes to five against to become associate members.

It was perhaps some small consolation to him that his students at the Polytechnic presented him with the original of a lithograph, made on chalkstone by Franz Schier (1815—1865) from a sketch by Anton Machek (1774—1844), signed by the two artists and inscribed "Dedicated in honour and gratitude from the class of 1839—1840 of the Prague Technical Institute" (page 35). This has since become the best known portrait of Doppler, published in many editions, one bearing the handwritten maxim which appears on page XIV.

In the meantime, the Dopplers' first son, Ludwig, had been born on 8th April 1838, to be followed almost exactly two years later by their second son, Adolf*, and in the same year (1840) they moved out of their accommodation in house number 4 on what is now the Charles Square *(Karlovo náměsti)* into the Long Avenue *(Dlouhá třída)*. It was therefore in this house that Doppler conceived and wrote the work that was to make him famous and not the house on the Charles Square as is suggested by the tablet that has been erected on it (see page 36).

By Imperial Decree of 6th March 1841, Doppler was appointed as full Professor of Elementary Mathematics and Practical Geometry at the Polytechnic Institute in Prague which apparently increased the already heavy burden of work he took upon himself. There are reports (13) of 800 students who Doppler must examine, with 668 written works to be read and classified by the increasingly sick Doppler, in addition to his duties within the Royal Bohemian Society of Sciences which Ivan Štoll, a successor of Doppler's at the Polytechnic (now the Czech Technical University), refers

* *It is of interest to note that on the Registration Form (page 49) this child is entered as "Gustav Adolf". The author can find no other record of this name ever being used.*

to as "the sunny side of Doppler's stay in Prague, which partly compensated his hardships, represented by his mostly speculative investigations in experimental physics. Overcoming his illness and exhaustion, he worked intensively, often during the night (night is after all the best time for the artist's and the scientist's concentration), suggesting new ideas and physical methods. He published a new optical method for measuring distances (the so-called diastemometer), discussed the aberration of light and sound in a rotating medium, recommended the application of photographic methods in astronomy, rediscovered the stroboscopic method (published earlier by Plateau and Stamper) but combined it with fog-horn and interrupted illumination, contemplated on the problems of electricity, undulations, geophysics, astronomy, etc." (84).

"On which of his works he placed the greatest value is difficult to say, at least for me", wrote Karl Kreil a few weeks after Doppler's death (56b), "since he seldom spoke about his work. Perhaps his favourites were those that were the most challenged, because they were those that became most widely known and to which he had most frequently to return. Had he ever possessed the gift not to send his ideas into the world as mere embryos, but to serve as their midwife, honing and forming them more for application, then recognition would probably have come more quickly."

It was at such a meeting of the Natural Sciences Section of the Royal Bohemian Society of Sciences, held in Prague on 25th May 1842 under the chairmanship of his friend and mentor Bernard Bolzano, that Doppler presented his work "On the Coloured Light of the Double Stars and Certain Other Stars of the Heavens" that was eventually to make his name known throughout the world. This appears in facsimile on pages 95—134, together with an English translation originally made in 1988 by my son and myself, which seems to be the first time that this milestone in scientific history had appeared in the English language (36). The original 1842 edition which was used for the facsimile is in the library of Salzburg University and is dedicated in Doppler's handwriting "From the author to the Imperial and Royal Lyceum Library as a gift". The university in Salzburg was dissolved by the Bavarians in 1810 and had the status of a Lyceum during Doppler's days there, and was not reinstated as a university until 1962.

How I came upon this priceless document in my search for Christian Doppler makes a rather amusing anecdote. My son and I had originally made our translation from a photocopy of a later version sent to us from the library of the University of Vienna. When I had the idea of publishing it in facsimile I went to the University Library in Salzburg to see if, by any

chance, there was a copy there. A check in the library catalogue confirmed that this was the case. After filling in the usual form to borrow this work it appeared on my library desk and my heart missed a beat as I opened the front page to see the dedication in Doppler's characteristic handwriting. No difficulty was experienced in taking it home (I lived in Germany at the time) to be photographed for the book and also, of course, to show it to a number of friends who had an interest in such a rare document. When my book containing this was published in November 1988, I presented one of the first copies to the Director of the University Library, dedicated "From the author, to the University Library in Salzburg as a gift". After thanking me, he added: "When you leave here I will telephone to have that Doppler work put on to the list of restricted books." Now, on the rare occasions that I like to have it — the most recent one being a visit by the President of Austria to our Christian Doppler exhibition in the Salzburg Science Museum — it is only with considerable difficulty and a great deal of form-filling that I can get my hands on it!

A few months after publication of the book, I was fortunate enough to have in my hands another priceless document which records one of the great events of science. Following an invitation from the Czechoslovakian Academy of Sciences, I made my first visit to Prague to lecture on the life and work of their illustrious ex-member. During my stay I was very kindly allowed to consult their archives. One of the first documents I sought was, naturally, the minutes of this famous meeting. It consists of an unprepossessing single sheet of brownish paper bearing a dozen lines of barely legible handwriting (page 37). The minute keeper, Johann Presl, was obviously not in his best form, as he had originally written the date as being 25th June 1842, and later crossed out the month to insert "May" over this. But the most remarkable revelation of this document, was to be informed that on the epoch making occasion, Doppler had, in addition to the minute keeper, only five listeners in his audience! It was also an exciting moment for me to visit the meeting room of the Royal Bohemian Academy of Sciences in the renowned Charles University (founded 1348) where Doppler probably presented his paper, although it is possible — particularly in view of the small number of participants — that the meeting was held in what is now the academic robing room nearby (47).

It is not my intention to give a critical assessment of Doppler's famous publication or his other work. For those interested, there are a number of such critiques (2, 43, 59, 89) but the most recent and thorough, by the Viennese physicist-writer Peter Schuster (42) is unfortunately at present only available in German. Suffice it to say here that Doppler's theory was not

based on any experimental observations of his own, but was a purely theoretical work encompassing the aberration theorum of Bradley (7) who he acknowledges in the sub-title of the paper and frequently throughout the work.

James Bradley was an Englishman who had been born some 150 years previously (March 1693). During his theological studies at Balliol College, Oxford, he developed a keen interest in astronomy, largely due to the influence of the eminent astronomer, Edmund Halley, who Bradley was later to succeed as Astronomer Royal. In 1721 Bradley resigned his position as Vicar of Bridstow to become Savilian Professor of Astronomy at Oxford University and in 1729 published "An Account of a new discovered motion of the fix'd Stars" in the form of a letter to Halley in the Philosophical Transactions of the Royal Society of London (7). This beautifully written account of how Bradley attempted to demonstrate the effect of parallax on the stars as the Earth rotated around the Sun, but finally attributed the abberations that he and others had observed as being due to the velocity of the observer on Earth, is a fine example of how erudition and perseverence could transform an early fallacy into a brilliant scientific success. My earlier reference to Bradley's letter as "the almost-Doppler principle" (32) is not as flippant as it might first appear!

Doppler commenced by reviewing the wave theory of light, by which colour perceived by the eye is dependent upon the frequency of the pulsations which stimulate it. Anything which changes the interval between these pulsations, changes the perceived colour. If the light source and the observer are both at rest, then the observed and the emitted frequency are the same. If the observer moves towards the source, however, the frequency will increase, and if he moves away it will decrease. Movement of the source will produce similar effects. Doppler used the analogy of a ship "steering towards the oncoming waves, which has to receive, in the same amount of time, more waves with a greater impact compared with a ship that is not moving or is even travelling along in the direction of the waves. If this should be valid for waves of water", he asked, "then why should it not also be applied — with necessary modifications — to air and ether waves?" (pages 108—109).

His paper ends with a final reference to Bradley and his "brilliant explanation of the phenomenon of aberration". "If a speed of 21.6 Miles (in the second) is sufficient to divert the direction of a beam of light by 20", then why should not a demonstrably greater speed produce a change in the colour and intensity of the light?" he asked (pages 130—131).

Although Doppler's general explanation of his theory and the supporting illustration he gave for sound were correct, the explanation and nine supporting arguments involving the changing colours of the stars (pages 114—117) were not. These were based on the fallacy that all stars emitted white light, and Doppler was also apparently unaware of the evidence of infrared and ultraviolet radiation which had been produced by Herschel (49) and Ritter (73) respectively some forty years earlier.

On 4th July 1843 the Doppler's fourth child, Bertha, was born in the house number 799 in what is now Court Lane *(u Obecního dvora)* to which they had moved (page 47). In the minutes of the Meeting of the Mathematical Section of the Royal Bohemian Society of Sciences held on 5th November 1843 we read:

"§ 7. On the occasion of the death on 1st November of the full member, Dr. Edler von Krombholz, the Secretary raised the question: 'Who should be given the responsibility of preparing his biography for the Annals of the Society?' At the request of the meeting Dr. Bolzano, as the oldest and closest friend of the deceased, took over this task."

"§ 8. At this point there began a discussion on the filling of the vacancy for a full member, which had now become available. In this respect the member Palacky proposed the associate member Doppler, to which proposal Bolzano and several other members agreed."

When these minutes were read at the next meeting of the Society (3rd December) the matter of Doppler's full membership was discussed and the vote was deferred to the next meeting. This was held on the last day of 1843 under the Chairmanship of Bolzano, with Kreil and Exner also being among the other ten members present. "Christian Doppler was elected as a Full Member of the Society by nine votes with one against", we can read in the minutes that are preserved in the archives of the Czechoslovakian Academy of Sciences, as is the letter sent by the Society on 15th January 1844 informing Doppler of his election. Towards the end of this year (12. 11. 1844) their fifth and last child, Hermann, was born.

These were Doppler's most productive years and he continued to publish most of his work in the Proceedings of the Royal Bohemian Society of Sciences. The first edition of his textbook on arithmetic and algebra was published in Prague in 1843 (18) with a second edition appearing in Vienna in 1851. But the academic year 1844—1845 was also a critical one for Doppler, with his respiratory disease being in an advanced stage, and his physi-

cian, Professor Johann von Oppolzer, advised him to give up his lectures "if he did not wish to meet his end as a result of consumption of the windpipe" (55). Only when he could not speak at all due to tuberculosis of the larynx (84) was he relieved of his duties, and we can read in the Annals of the Polytechnic Institute for 1845 that his lectures were taken over by Joseph John.

A critical article on his theory by the well-known astronomer Mädler which appeared in the newspaper *Stuttgarter Morgenblatt* was thoroughly refuted by Doppler in a lengthy article which he published in the Austrian Pages for Literature and Art (19). He had firstly sent this rebuttal to the editor of the Stuttgart newspaper who declined to publish such an extensive reply, Doppler remarked in a footnote.

In the Summer of 1844, under an ever increasing work load, (according to his grandson, he remarked ironically to his friend Franz Exner at this time that, after completing his work for the Royal Society, he would examine 500 students "for relaxation") he began these examinations too early and only in the written form, so hat he could hurry away to Salzburg on 11th July to seek treatment for his rapidly deteriorating condition. Angry parents also protested that his classification of the results was far too hard. These results were therefore invalidated by the authorities and an enquiry was held.

This minor scandal, and its effect on the sensitive and introverted Doppler, made him decide to leave Prague as quickly as possible. Franz Exner informed him of a vacant position as manager of a cotton-spinning factory, to which Doppler spontaneously responded with great enthusiasm in a letter dated 29th September 1845, only to realise more soberly a few days later that he was not really intended to be a manager.

At about this time a remarkable work on the Doppler effect was published by a young Dutchman who had just obtained his doctorate from the University of Utrecht, Christoph Hendrik Diederik Buys Ballot. This son of a Dutch reformed pastor — and himself a lay preacher — did not believe that Doppler's theory could explain the coloured light of the double stars and decided that it should be put to the test. This he proclaimed in Latin at the beginning of a scientific work published in 1845 (9). Since no practical experimental conditions existed in those days for attaining the high speeds required to test a source of light, Buys Ballot's experiments were restricted to a rapidly moving source of sound. Fortunately for him, the railway between Utrecht and Amsterdam had been completed two years previously

and he was able to persuade the Dutch government to put this at his disposal, together with a locomotive capable of attaining speeds of 40 miles per hour and a flat-car for his experiments.

For the first experiment on the stretch between Utrecht and Maarsen in February 1845, Buy Ballot had horn-players posted along the track and also riding on the railway car. Unfortunately, the winter weather caused continual interruptions, and snow and hailstorms resulted in the musicians not being able to blow their instruments properly (52)! The experiments were therefore postponed to the more clement weather of June and were conducted on a somewhat more sophisticated scale, involving teams of musicians with previously calibrated instruments, musically trained observers and Buys Ballot himself riding on the footplate of the locomotive. It was observed that, as the locomotive passed the players stationed on each side of the track, the note blown by the musicians on the train was perceived half a tone higher as it approached and half a tone lower as it receded. In other words, the validity of Doppler's theory was confirmed, but Buys Ballot was still sceptical about its application to light.

Doppler's chance to leave Prague, which he had been trying to do since 1837, came early in 1847 when a professorship in mathematics, physics and mechanics became available at the Academy of Mining and Forestry in Schemnitz (today Banská Štiavnica).

Christian Doppler.
Lithograph by Franz Schier (Sir) from a sketch by Anton Machek.

(Reproduced by kind permission of the picture archives of the Austrian National Library, Vienna)

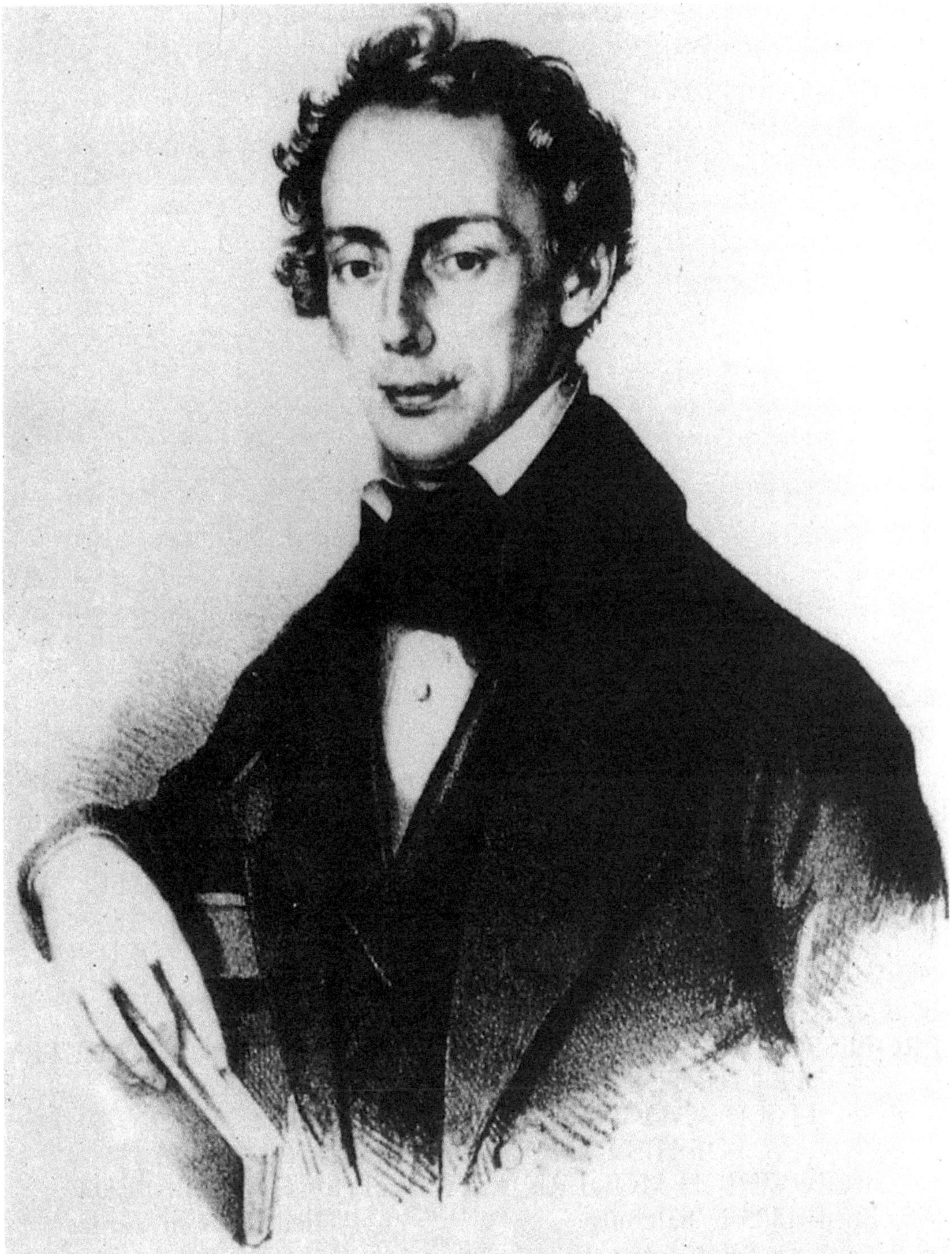

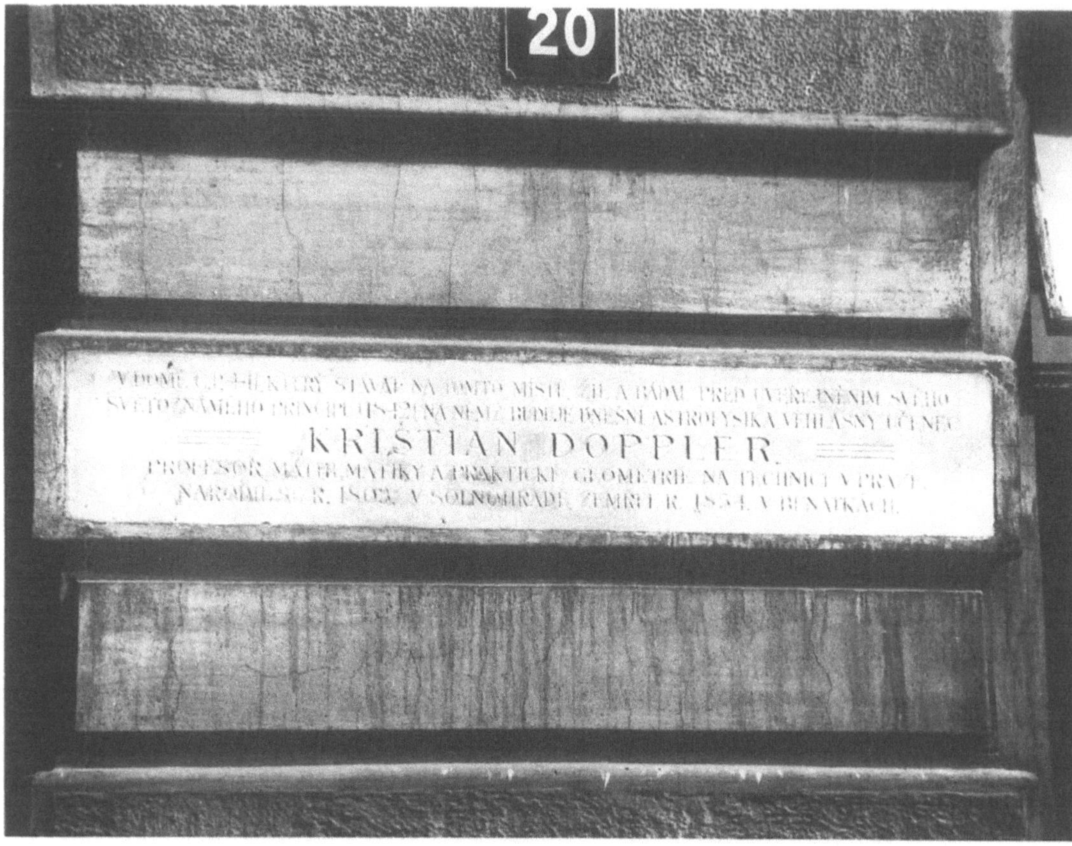

A commemorative tablet erected on a courthouse on the Charles Square in Prague on the 100th anniversary of Christian Doppler's birthday. It reads:

IN HOUSE NO: 4/II WHICH STOOD ON THIS SITE
THE RENOWNED SCIENTIST

CHRISTIAN DOPPLER

PROFESSOR OF MATHEMATICS AND PRACTICAL GEOMETRY
AT THE TECHNICAL INSTITUTE OF PRAGUE
LIVED AND WORKED ON THE PUBLICATION
OF HIS FAMOUS PRINCIPLE (1842)
ON WHICH MODERN ASTROPHYSICS ARE BASED
Born: 1803 in Salzburg Died: 1854 in Venice

The year of death (1853) is incorrectly stated, and it is seen from the official Registration Form of the Doppler family (page 49) that they moved out of this house already in 1840.

(Photograph by the author)

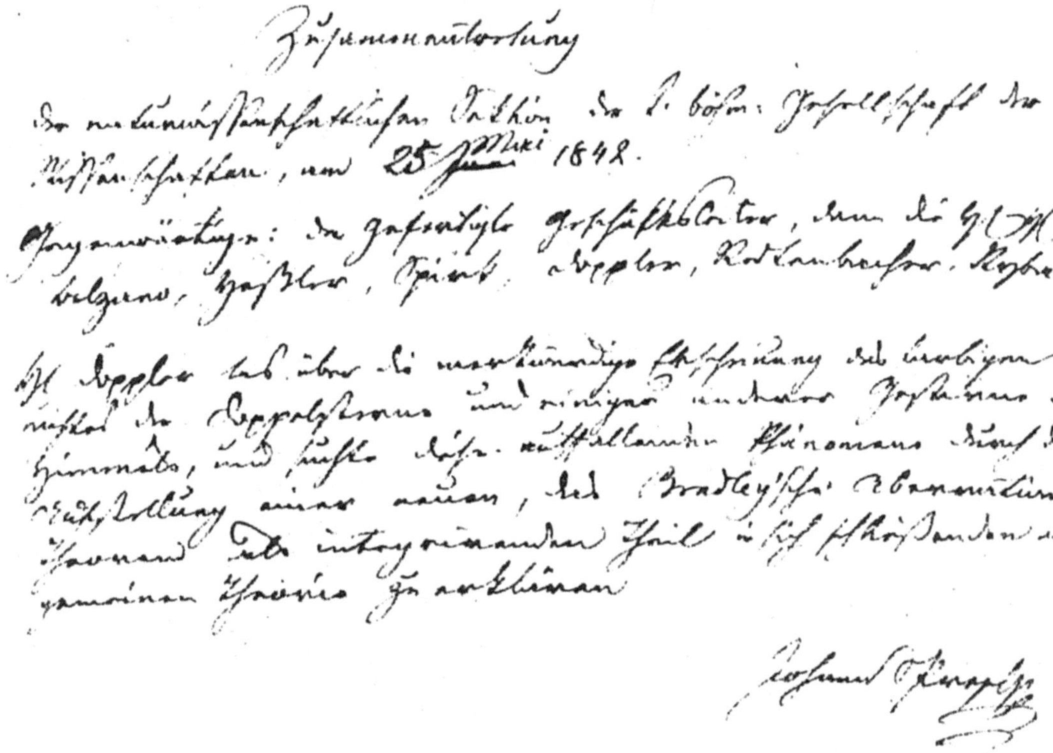

Minutes of the meeting of the Natural Sciences Section of the Royal Bohemian Society of Sciences held on 25th May 1842 in Prague. It reads:

1842, 25 May

Meeting

of the Natural Sciences Section of the Royal Bohemian Society of Sciences on 25th May 1842.

Present: the keeper of the minutes, then the members Bolzano, Hessler, Spirk, Doppler, Redtenbacher, Ryba.

Doppler read on the strange appearance of the coloured light of the double stars and certain other stars of the heavens and attempted to explain this noticable phenomenon by putting forward a new theory which includes Bradley's aberration theorem as an integral part of a general theory.

Johann Presl

(With kind permission of the Archives of the Czechoslovakian Academy of Sciences, Prague)

The Doppler Family

Doppler spent more than twelve years in Prague, during which time he not only produced the majority and the most famous of his scientific works, but also married a devoted wife who bore him five children during their stay in the golden city. It is therefore not out of place here to take a brief look at Christian Doppler, not so much as a scientist, but as a family man and father.

He had been in Prague little more that a year when he returned to Salzburg to marry Mathilde, the daughter of Franz Sturm, a gold and silversmith in that city. As with so much of Doppler's biographical data, there is some confusion about the date of their marriage. During a special commemorative session of the Imperial Academy of Sciences in Vienna, held on 30th May 1853 to mark Doppler's death two months previously, the general secretary, Professor Anton Schrötter (80), gives the date as 11th April 1836. This was based on the opening sentence of a letter dated 12th May 1853 (now in the archives of the Austrian Academy of Sciences in Vienna (56b)) from the astronomer Karl Kreil, who was not only a contemporary of Doppler in Prague and Vienna, but was also later to become the brother-in-law of Dr. Hermann von Pflügl of Linz, who married Doppler's eldest daughter Mathilde. Doppler's grandson Adolf, on the other hand, gives the date simply as "February 1836" (14). In a recently published historical work on Christian Doppler in the German language, Grössing and Schuster (42) give the first date in one part of their biography but follow the example of Adolf Doppler in a later section on the Doppler family, giving the more precise date of 11th February 1836 without any account for this apparent discrepancy. A check of the original record of the marriage performed by the Benedictine Father Michael Filz at the Church of Mülln in Salzburg which is now in the Consistorial Archives of that city confirms that 11th April is the correct date.

Mathilde Doppler was described by Karl Kreil (56) who knew the family well, as being "more of a domesticated nature, although in this respect and as a mother commendable to the highest degree, she did not understand his scientific thoughts". Professor Karel Kořistka, who was Doppler's assistant in Schemnitz in 1848, described her as being "of a still, deep nature" (77).

Christian Doppler was of a rather shy, introverted and sensitive character. His thrifty nature, which enabled him to survive on a minimal income as an assistant in Vienna at the time of his father's death, was referred to by his

mother in 1830 at a session of the civil court to decide on the inheritance of her late husband (29). It was a characteristic which also enabled him to support a large family on the modest income of a professor in later life, largely by turning his back on the social life of Prague and Vienna. Despite this, he lived in almost continual trepidation of not being able to maintain a family of seven, and complained bitterly at the rising prices in Prague.

He was a man of few friends. One exception in Prague was the philosopher and mathematician Bernard Bolzano, who was relieved of his offices as priest and professor of religion in 1819 because of his non-conformist teachings (39). It was Bolzano who proposed Doppler for membership of the Royal Bohemian Society of Sciences (4) and who had chaired the meeting at which he presented his famous theory, which he supported in his publications (5, 6). A further friend during the last years of Doppler's life was Franz Exner, the philosopher and educational reformist who was largely responsible for Doppler's appointment to the chair of experimental physics in Vienna. Exner accompanied Doppler to Venice in November 1852 and died in Padua three months after Doppler's death. Due to this lack of close friends, there is practically no correspondence from Doppler that gives us a deeper insight into his character. Besides his modesty and correctness, the one quality upon which virtually all contemporaries and biographers of Doppler are agreed is his extreme industriousness and capacity for hard work despite the illness that dogged him for most of his life.

"Doppler was of a tall lean build, already showing signs of the respiratory illness that was to result in his early death", Karel Kořistka commented on his earlier director. "He had the nature of a true scholar, quiet and friendly, living only for science. His large bright eyes signalled a spirit which by far outshone the normal" (77).

As we have seen, Christian Doppler also wrote poetry and essays, at least in his earlier years, and we learn from his grandson Adolf that he also showed great skill in cutting silhouettes from paper — indeed, he had planned to support himself from this dexterity during his initial period in America that almost came to be in 1834. His musical talent on the flute is also reported by his grandson (but see footnote on page 15!).

The family portrait on page 46 is from a daguerreotype probably made by Wilhelm Horn in 1844. The glass plates were partially restored in 1903 so that the head and shoulders of Christian Doppler could be used by Dr. Karl Haas to illustrate the lecture he had given to celebrate the 100th an

niversary of Doppler's birth when this was printed in the Quarterly Report of the Viennese Society for the Furtherance of Physical and Chemical Teaching the following year under the title "Christian Doppler and his Discoveries" (43).

The two older children on each side of the group appear to be leaning on their parents, while the smallest child in the middle is firmly wedged between his mother and father. This is due to the fact that it was necessary to sit motionless for periods of up to an hour for the exposure of such a daguerreotype in those days. It is for this reason that the Doppler's youngest child, Bertha, who would have been about one year old at the time of this portrait, is not in the picture. What cannot be seen is that Professor and Mrs. Doppler are almost certainly leaning on wooden headrests to give them some support during this long sitting.

Mathilde Doppler is obviously in an advanced stage of pregnancy with her last child, Hermann, who was born in November 1844. It is this fact that helps us to date this portrait so accurately. In August 1881 Hermann was to marry Maria Liebscher who bore him five children, one who was called Christian Doppler who died in 1938, and another who was Dr. Adolf Doppler (died 1969, aged 85 years) from whom we have so much information on his grandfather. Neither of these two sons, nor the three daughters, ever married and this line of the Doppler family died out with the death of Hermine Doppler in Vienna on 15th June 1975.

Bertha, the missing daughter in the portrait, married in Vienna at the age of almost 35 to Lieutenant-Colonel Otto Edler von Klein. There were two sons and a daughter from this marriage, and one of the sons, the lawyer Dr. Gustav von Klein-Doppler, adopted the hyphenated names of his parents. It is his daughter, Dorothea Merstallinger, Christian Doppler's great granddaughter who lives in retirement just outside of Vienna. Frau Merstallinger has been a valuable source of information in my search for Christian Doppler and has most generously donated several items of Doppler memorabilia to the Christian Doppler Foundation in Salzburg, including the original glass plates of the daguerreotype portrait illustrated here. It was indeed a memorable moment for me, on the anniversary of Doppler's death in March 1990, to be present with Frau Merstallinger, her son and her nephew, in Venice for the unveiling of the commemorative tablet on the house in which Doppler died and to lay a wreath on his memorial (page 76).

The 4 year-old child jammed between his parents is Adolf, who was to become one of Austria's most famous engineers for which he received a knighthood. Adolf von Doppler (died 24. 6. 1916 in Vienna, aged 76) married Minna Unger from Hannover who bore him two daughters, both of whom died without children.

Ludwig, on the left of the picture, was the eldest son and would have been six years old at the time of this portrait. He took up a military career and died in 1906 without marrying.

The eldest child, who leans on her father, was named Mathilde after her mother and became the second wife of a medical practitioner from Linz, Dr. Hermann von Pflügl. Their only child Alfred (1863—1929) was an artist who had a son (who died at the age of 26) and also a daughter, Mathilda Anna Emilia Sophie von Pflügl, now living in Rio de Janeiro, Brazil. It was Frau von Pflügl who donated to the Austrian Academy of Sciences the portrait of her great grandfather shown on page 44. The twin portrait of Mathilde Doppler is in her possession.

When this portrait of the Doppler family was made in 1844, they were living on the first floor of house number 799 in the *Hofgasse* (Court Lane) shown on page 47. They lived in this house, in which Hermann was born, until they left Prague in 1847. This was Doppler's sixth residence in Prague and was just a stone's throw away from their previous house (No. 922) in what is now the Long Avenue *(Dluohá třída)*. Previous to this they had lived in the House No. 4 in the 2nd district which is now the site of the court building on the Charles Square which bears the misleading commemorative plaque shown on page 36.

Christian Doppler's first home in Prague was House No. 146 in the *v Jirchářich* just off the Island Street *(Ostrovní)* was probably a one-room bachelor accommodation from which he had to move into House No. 22 in what is now *Jungmannova třída* when his newlywed wife joined him in 1836. It is also possible, particularly in view of Doppler's pronounced thriftiness referred to earlier, that the Dopplers moved each time there was an addition to the family. The official registration form on page 49 does not give us the dates of moving from the earlier residences, but the two last moves (1840 and 1843) certainly correspond with the birth of their last two children.

Their final move from Prague was made at the end of 1847, when their five children ranged in age from barely three years to almost ten.

Christian Andreas Doppler

An oil painting on wood made by an unknown artist, probably in 1836 at the time of his marriage. The original is in the possession of the Austrian Academy of Sciences, to whom it was donated in 1976 by Mathilda von Pflügl of Rio de Janeiro, the great granddaughter of Christian Doppler. The corresponding portrait of **Mathilde Doppler** née Sturm (opposite) is still in Rio de Janeiro. These photographs were made from copies generously donated to the Christian Doppler Foundation by its vice president, Professor Gunther Ladurner.

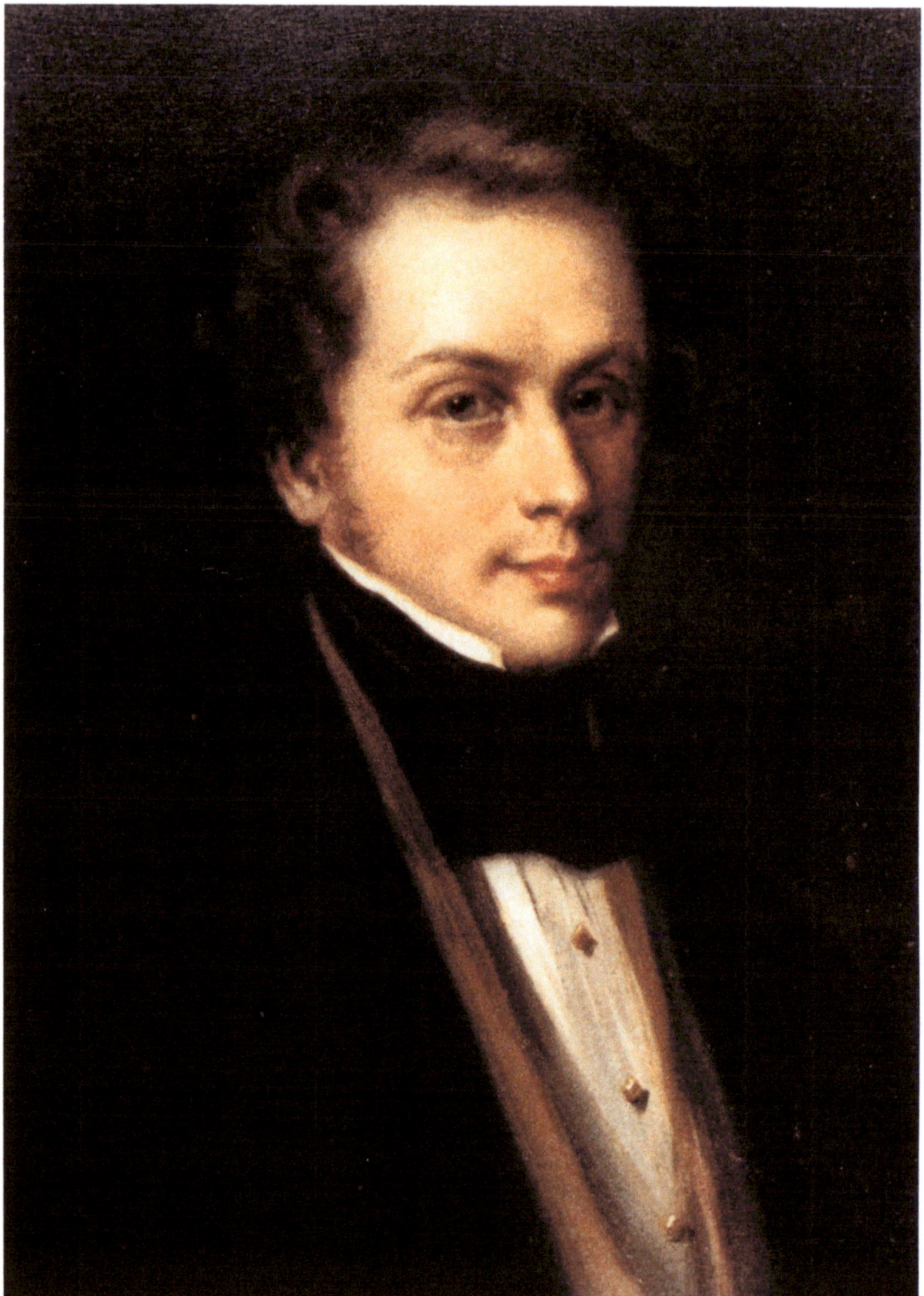

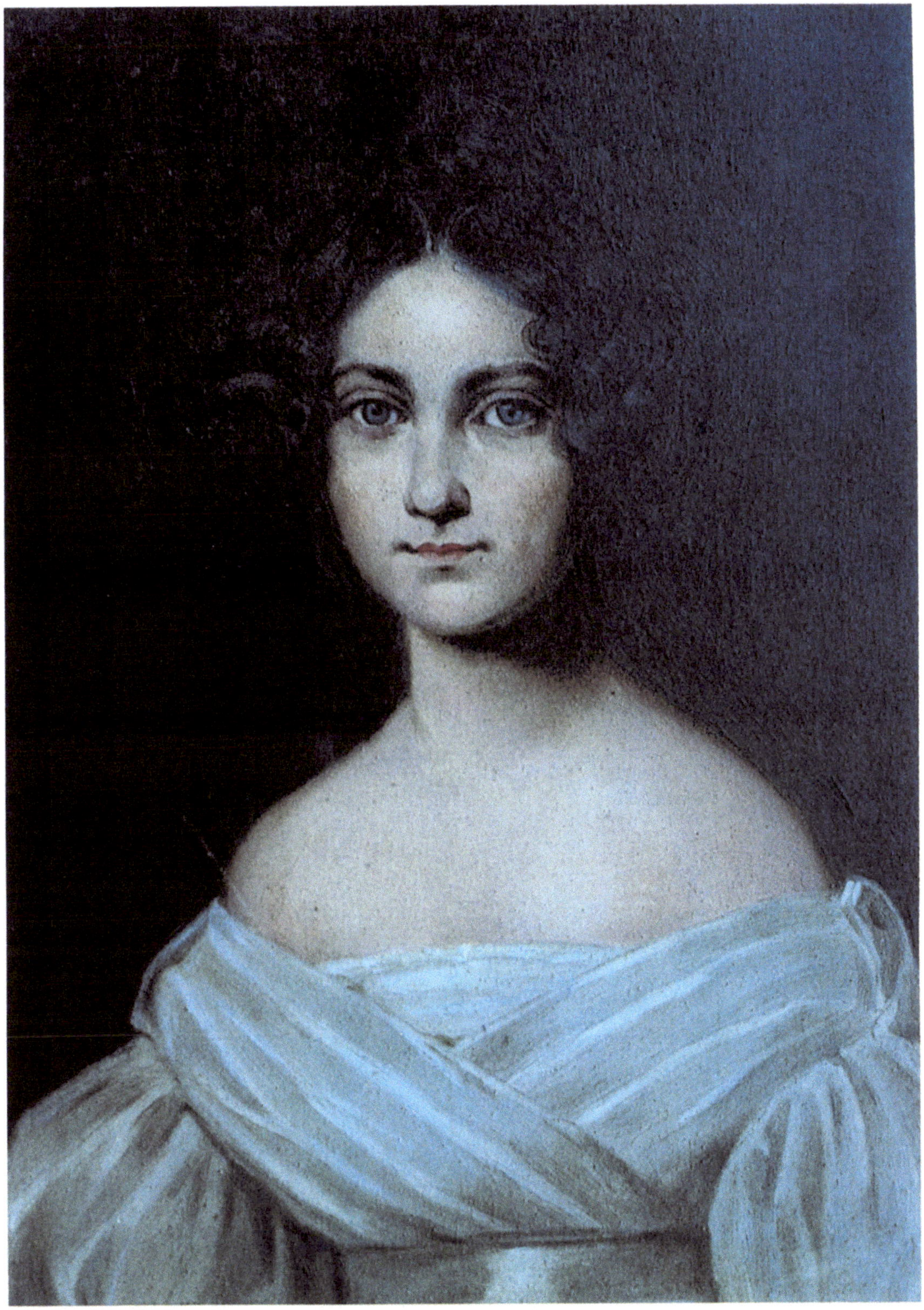

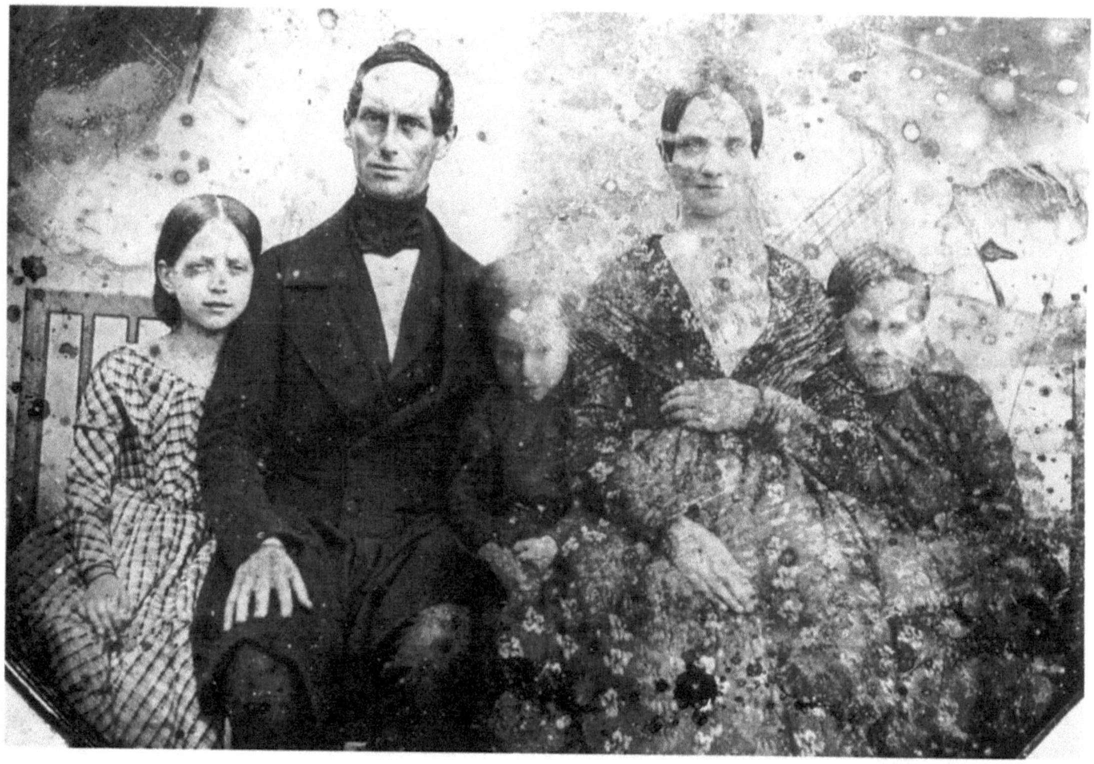

The Doppler Family

Daguerreotype by Wilhelm Horn of Prague 1840
For a detailed description see pages 40—42.

(Original glass plates generously donated to the Christian Doppler Foundation by Frau Dorothea Merstallinger, great granddaughter of Christian Doppler)

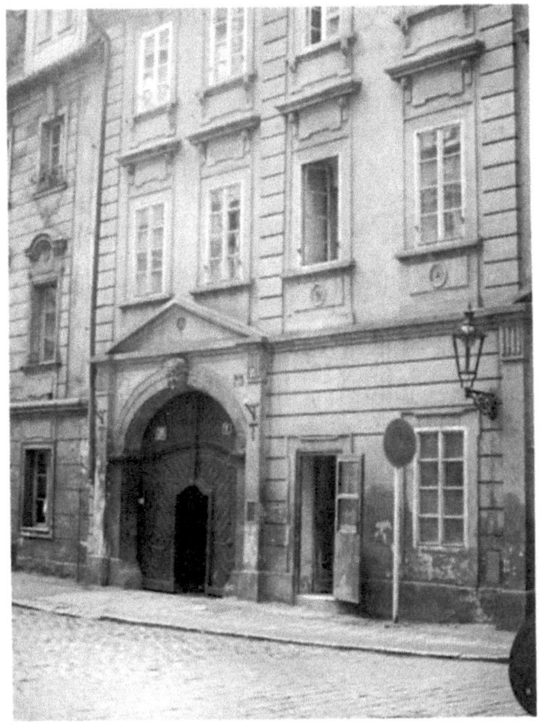

House No: 799 in the *Hofgasse* in Prague. The Doppler Family lived on the first floor from 1843 until they left the city in 1847.

(Photograph by the author)

Detail from the registration form *(Konscriptionsbogen)* of the Doppler Family in Prague. It lists the names of Christian Doppler, his wife Mathilde, the sons Ludwig, Gustav Adolf and Hermann, followed by their daughters Mathilde and Bertha, giving the years of their birth. On the left are the numbers of the six houses in which they lived during their twelve years in the city.

Opposite Doppler's name is written: "Professor of Mathematics at the State Secondary School. Born in Salzburg. Married." Above the list of names: "According to decree No 154 of 13th January 1836 from the Director of the State Technical Institute, remunerated with 1000 Florins."

(With kind permission of the State Archives in Prague)

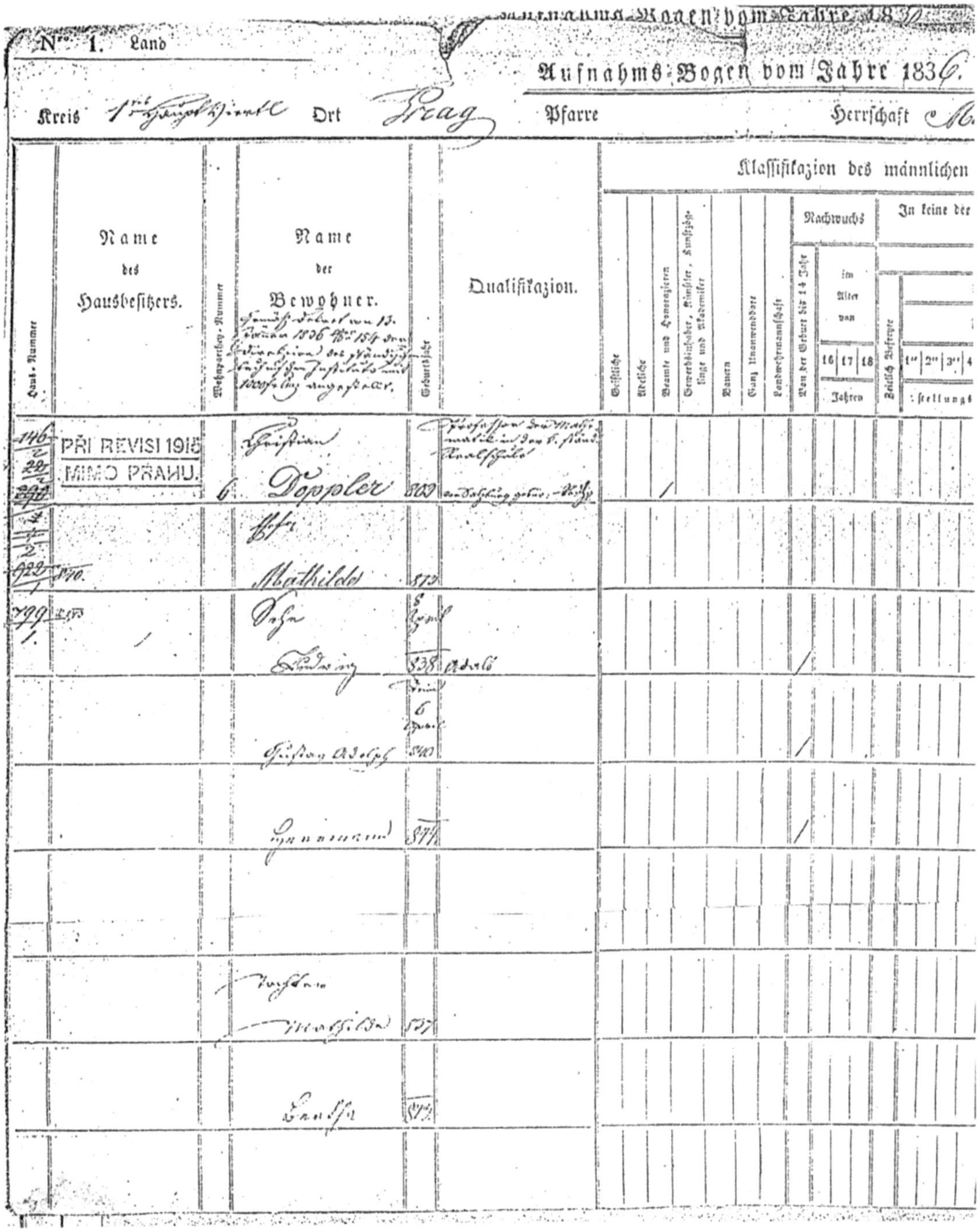

Nro. 1. Land

Aufnahms-Bogen vom Jahre 1836.

Kreis 1ter Hauptbezirk Ort Prag Pfarre Herrschaft M.

Haus-Nummer	Name des Hausbesitzers.	Wohnparthey-Nummer	Name der Bewohner.	Geburtsjahr	Qualifikazion.	Geistliche	Adeliche	Beamte und Honoratioren	Gewerbsinhaber, Künstler, Kunstzöglinge und Akademiker	Bauern	Ganz Unanwendbare	Landwehrmannschaft	Von der Geburt bis 14 Jahr	Nachwuchs im Alter von 16	17	18 Jahren	Zeitlich Befreyte	In keine der … 1"/2"/3"/4 … stellungs
146 / 2 / 22 / 299	PŘI REVISI 1915 MIMO PRAHU.	6	Christian Doppler	803	Professor der Mathematik an der ständ. Realschule; anderhalbjährig …			1										
4 / 1 / 2 / 922 / 1	1840		Ehefr. Mathilde	813														
799 / 1	1873		Sohn Ludwig	838									1					
			Gustav Adolph	6 April 840									1					
			Hermann	844									1					
			Tochter Mathilde	837														
			Bertha	844														

1848: A Turbulent Interlude

By an Imperial Decree of 23rd October 1847 Doppler was appointed as Professor of Mathematics and Mechanics at the Academy of Mining and Forestry in Schemnitz, which was then in the Hungarian part of the Austrian Empire and is today Banská Štiavnica in Czechoslovakia. The mining academy enjoyed an excellent reputation throughout Europe and Doppler certainly improved himself financially as a result of this move. We know from his letter of appointment dated 11th November 1847, which is now in the city archives of Prague, that Doppler received an annual salary of 1,500 Florins, which was an increase of 100 Florins over his last salary in Prague. In addition, he had the right to official living quarters or an annual allowance of 150 Florins, as well as an allowance of 116 Florins yearly for fuel and lighting. This meant an overall increase of about 25 % of his income.

The Doppler family moved into one of the official living quarters of the Academy, probably on the second floor of the *Belházy* house which had been vacant since 1843 (69).

On 11th December 1847 Doppler took his oath as professor, which contained passages that already reflected the political tension existing prior to the revolution of 1848—1849. He had to swear that if anything should come to his attention "that could threaten the welfare and rights of His Majesty, to report this without delay to the responsible authorities and not be drawn into any machinations". "Do you swear", he was challenged, "that you do not belong to any secret society, neither at home nor abroad? If you do belong to such an organisation, then leave it immediately, and do not join such societies in the future."

At the beginning of 1848 Karel Kořistka came to Schemnitz as Doppler's assistant and we are told (77) that this was a most pleasant relationship, with Doppler treating him like a son. From him we also learn of Doppler's annoyance at the political unrest in Hungary, under which his calm and scholarly nature suffered considerably. He complained that he could no longer bear this and arranged to be on holiday during the summer semester, appointing Kořistka to supplement in his absence, and did not return until the autumn. But the turmoil increased. The Hungarian uprising broke out and the army of insurrection occupied all mining cities, hoping to find supplies of gold and silver. The Imperial Army then besieged and bombarded Schemnitz.

According to a story told to Adolf Doppler by his uncle (Christian Doppler's son Adolf, who would have been nine years old at the time), which is largely supported by Kořistka, the commandant of the revolutionary army, Artur von Görgey, heard of Doppler's presence in Schemnitz and sought him out for a discussion. He knew Doppler from his days in Prague where he had studied chemistry from 1846 to 1848. Doppler was apparently not too happy about meeting with the revolutionary leader and insisted that the conversation should be confined to scientific matters and by no means touch on politics. He asked Karel Kořistka to be present as a witness to this. We are told that the night was taken up with lively scientific discussion amidst the noise of the bombardment, during which von Görgey suggested that they should test Foucault's pendulum experiments in one of the disused mineshafts in Schemnitz (42).

It is characteristic of Christian Doppler that he would not allow the turmoil of the Hungarian uprising — in addition to his already failing health — to deter him from his scientific works, four of which he published during 1848. Just a few weeks after leaving Schemnitz he presented a paper, at a meeting of the Imperial Academy of Sciences in Vienna on 14th April 1849, "On an as yet unused source of magnetic declination observations" which was based on his work in this mining city, where the many underground tunnels had inspired him with the idea of measuring changes in the magnetic declination which had been entered on to old maps. Such changes represent an extremely complex physical phenomenon which, although reportedly observed by the Chinese in the 8th Century, is still not fully understood today (65). In the following year Doppler was to publish three important works on this subject.

It was against this turbulent background that two great honours were bestowed upon Christian Doppler. On 26th January 1848 he was elected as a full member of the Imperial Academy of Sciences in Vienna and his election was confirmed on 1st February. In the same year he was awarded an honorary doctorate in philosophy by the Charles University in Prague which was celebrating the 500th anniversary of its foundation*. The official ceremony, originally planned to be held on 28th August 1848 in that historic building where Doppler had presented his famous work six years earlier, was at first postponed due to the unrest and demonstrations that

* *Curiously enough, he was also proposed for an honorary doctorate by the medical faculty (47), which today would certainly be justifiable, but it is difficult to understand on what grounds it was proposed at the time. In any event, it was decided that the honorary doctorate in philosophy would be more fitting.*

were also taking place in Prague and was eventually abandoned. The doctoral certificate was not sent to Doppler and the others being honoured until March 1849 (47).

Also in 1848 the engineer of the Great Eastern Railway in Britain, Scott Russell (76) published the results of his experiments in which he observed the significant difference between the tone of a locomotive's whistle and that reflected from the wall of the tunnel through which it passed at high speed. This was a most graphic demonstration of the Doppler shift, but Scott Russell did not give one word of credit to Doppler. "He either did not know about Doppler's work — or he did not want to know", said the Secretary General of the Imperial Academy of Sciences in Vienna in eulogising its famous member shortly after his death (80).

On 20th December 1848 Doppler was appointed as the successor to the retired Simon Stampfer at the Polytechnic Institute in Vienna. Due to the postal delays caused by the revolutionary activities, Doppler replied only on 8th February 1849 accepting the position. From the archives of the Technical University in Vienna, we learn that he arrived in Vienna on 24th February to take up his appointment.

The Return to Vienna

On their return to Vienna, the Doppler family moved into accommodation in the *Paniglgasse* (House No. 54) close to the Technical University where Christian Doppler became Professor of Practical Geometry on the retirement of the man who had launched him on his scientific career, Simon Stampfer. His tenure in this position, however, was to be less than a year. On 17th January 1850, the Emperor Franz Joseph signed a letter of appointment (page 61) authorising the foundation of an Institute of Physics at the Imperial University in Vienna, with Doppler as its first Director and Professor of Experimental Physics in the Philosophical Faculty there. Less than three months after his forty-sixth birthday, Doppler had reached the pinnacle of his academic career.

Doppler's appointment to this important position resulted from the reforms in higher education being instituted by the Imperial Minister of Culture and Education, Count Leo Thun-Hohenstein, whose State Secretary was Franz Exner. It was probably the influence of this good friend of Doppler's which helped to secure him this professorship in the face of strong competition from Andreas von Ettingshausen, who had held the Chair of Physics at the Imperial University since 1834, having previously been Professor of Higher Mathematics at the same seat of learning.

Certainly in a proposal of the Minister to Emperor Franz Joseph dated 1st December 1849 the words of Exner are clearly evident. "Concerning the direction of the Institute, I am in the position to draw to your attention to a man whose capabilities for this office have already been shown in a brilliant manner, despite the limited support he has so far received, and whose genius would now be given the opportunity to fully develop in this position." In proposing Doppler, reference is made to his "more than sixty scientific works in the publications of the learned society of Prague and the Viennese Academy of Sciences", although we can only find records of about 40 publications in any journals at this time. A little further in this proposal we learn that "he has repeatedly received offers from foreign universities as professor of physics, which he has, however, declined out of love for his fatherland". Grössing (42) points out that this is also somewhat exaggerated since, besides the offer from Bern in 1834 which was from a secondary school, his grandson talks only of an undefined offer from Switzerland in 1835 (which may have been that from Bern) and another for the Chair in Physics from the University of Marburg in 1848.

Doppler's position at the Technical University was taken over by his assistant, Anton Stampfer (possibly a son of Simon Stampfer who had recognised Doppler's talents already in his youth), and on 21st January 1850 Christian Doppler swore his oath as a professor at the Imperial University. His institute was firstly located under very cramped conditions in the Institute of Physics at the university, which had hardly recovered from its occupation by the student army (The Academic Legion) in March 1848 during the uprising of that stormy year. Since 1857 this magnificent building has been the home of the Austrian Academy of Sciences on the *Ignaz-Seipel-Platz*, but the Viennese still tend to refer to this as the *Universitätsplatz* and the building as the "Old University". It was here in August 1850 that Johann Gregor Mendel took a written and oral examination in the hope of entering the university. Doppler's judgement of the 28 year-old Augustinian monk who was later to lay the foundations of genetics was not very positive. "This essay", he reportes, "makes it clear that the candidate is formally well educated, but in the physical sciences, however, has not progressed beyond the elementary stage" (11). Other examiners were even less positive and Mendel did not obtain his entrance to the university until the following year.

Doppler's time was largely taken up with obtaining funds for the purchase of equipment and the recruitment of personnel as well as the setting up of a library there. He was at last becoming a manager! He also had to look for a new building to house his institute, which he found in the Viennese suburb of Erdberg — house number 104 in the *Hauptstrasse*, which later became *Erdbergstrasse* No. 15 (page 62)*. The upper two floors of this house provided ample room to fulfill its new role and had a large garden at the rear where, under the horse chestnut trees, large scale experiments could be carried out. Professor and Mrs. Doppler were to live with their five children in the apartment under the roof. Doppler himself negotiated a lease with the owner, Herr Klier (25), in the spring of 1851 and had hoped to move his institute and his family there in the summer, but his health had so deteriorated that he requested to take holiday from 16th July, and the Ministry of Education gave him permission to take sick-leave for the entire summer vacation, probably in Salzburg. So the move was delayed until the autumn and it was not until 10th October 1851 that the Philosophical Faculty could report to the University Consistory that Professor Doppler and his laboratory assistant, Joseph Riedl, had taken up residence in their official quarters.

* *This building was badly damaged by bombs in the Second World War and was only temporarily repaired. In 1986 it was completely demolished and now only the horse chestnut trees stand sadly in a car park.*

Students, including Gregor Mendel who had now matriculated at the university, received two hours daily instruction "in demonstrative and experimental physics from the Professor and Director of the Institute of Physics, Dr. Christian Doppler, in the Institute building: Erdberg, Hauptstrasse No. 104". In this unusually mild winter they also carried out some experiments in the garden to determine the pressure of steam by means of a specially constructed siren and flywheel (24), which were prompted by a series of explosions that had occured on the Austrian railways.

"The institute that was then housed in Erdberg was proof that significant achievements can be made in bad accommodation", the physicist Zemantsek in quoted as saying (12). "Yes, Erdberg remained with me for the rest of my life as a symbol of serious, cerebral experimental activity. When I was successful in bringing some life into the Institute of Physics in Graz, I called this jokingly 'little Erdberg'. Not little in space, since it was perhaps twice as large. But I had not for a long time come under the spell of the Erdberg spirit. Not in Munich, where the young doctors came to me wanting to work, only they didn't know on what? I thought: In Erdberg we were other persons. Here the most beautiful equipment stands around and we wonder what we can do with it. We always had more than enough ideas, only our problem was where to get the apparatus."

Doppler's teaching duties were increasingly taken over by his assistant Pekarek. His health had reached a low ebb and he was continually being urged by his medical adviser to take sick leave in the milder climate of the south. Added to this, his theory — and his reputation — were being attacked by a fellow member of the Imperial Academy of Sciences, Josef Petzval, who was Professor of Mathematics and Mechanics at the Imperial University. The arena for these attacks was the meetings at the Academy of Sciences in Vienna and there can be no doubt that Petzval was the aggressor (41). The temperamental dispute was carried out in a heated manner that was seldom experienced in the meetings of the Academy, which were normally noted for their factual scientific discussion.

Petzval's objections to Doppler's theory were based on a gross overestimation of the role of higher mathematics. In his work "On a general principle of undulation theory: the law of maintenance of the wavelength" (67) with which he responded to Doppler's theory at a meeting of the Academy of Sciences on 15th January 1852, Petzval stated that it was not possible to present much of value in a study of eight pages based only on simple equations. "Without the application of differential equations, it is not possible to enter the realms of great science."

In these objections Petzval confused two completely different cases: one in which there is relative movement between the sound source and the listener, and the other in which the medium is in motion but the sound source and listener are stationary. In the second case there is, according to the Doppler principle, no change in tone. In fact, Petzval's protracted and hard attacks, which came to a head during the meeting of the Academy of Sciences under the presidency of Andreas von Baumgartner on 21st May 1852, were eventually shown to be the best mathematical proof of Doppler's theory.

The minutes of this meeting in the archives of the Austrian Academy of Sciences tell us soberly that "the full member, Prof. Petzval held a lecture 'On the unsuitability of certain popular ways of looking at the undulation theory and their inability to replace the principle of maintenance of the wavelength'. He presented the manuscript for the report on the meeting (68). The full member, Professor Doppler, hereupon read a note entitled 'Remarks on the essays: on a general principle of the undulation theory' and presented this for the report on the meeting (26). The full member Director von Ettingshausen also read some remarks on the essay referred to which are also intended for the report." (38)

An interesting insight into this academic struggle is given in Egon von Opplzer's speech at the unveiling of the bust of Doppler in the colonnades of Vienna University in 1901 (63). "His opponent bandied with such expressions as 'great science' and 'small science' in the Academy of Sciences, being of the opinion that great truths could not be found in a few lines and through an equation with only one unknown, and that at least one differential equation is necessary — and in this way he believes to have shown the incorrectness of the Doppler principle. Whoever probes somewhat deeper will find in these attacks, not a purly scientific motive, but a more personal goal. It is the old contradiction between genius and talent which must lead to a struggle when, on the side of the talent there is no understanding of intuitive action and individual brilliance. For Doppler, surveying his principle, it is of clear certainty, and for him — a true natural researcher — the attack on a law that has already been confirmed through experiments is completely incomprehensible. He responded in a factual and decisive manner."

Doppler's "remarks" on Petzval's essay (26) and one further defence against Petzval's attack (27) were to be his last scientific publications. On 29th October 1852 the Minister of Education granted Doppler a six-months period of convalescence in the Kingdom of Lombardy-Venice from

1st November. He was accompanied on his journey by his good friend and fellow academician, Franz Exner, who was to die three months after Doppler. The directorship of the Institute of Physics was temporarily transferred to von Ettingshausen. This appointment was made permanent by a decree dated 25th November 1852, which also removed Doppler from his post. It ended: "The future capacity of Professor Doppler will be regulated following the restoration of his health."

Doppler's Letter of Appointment from the Emperor Franz Joseph.
It reads:

I authorise the foundation of an Institute of Physics as an integral part of the Faculty of Philosophy at the University of Vienna, following the proposal of my Minister of Culture and Education, and I appoint as Director of this Institute and to full Professor of Experimental Physics, the Professor of Practical Geometry at the Polytechnic Institute, Dr. Christian Doppler.

Vienna, 17th January 1850 Franz Joseph

(Reproduced by kind permission of the Central Library of the Institute of Physics, University of Vienna)

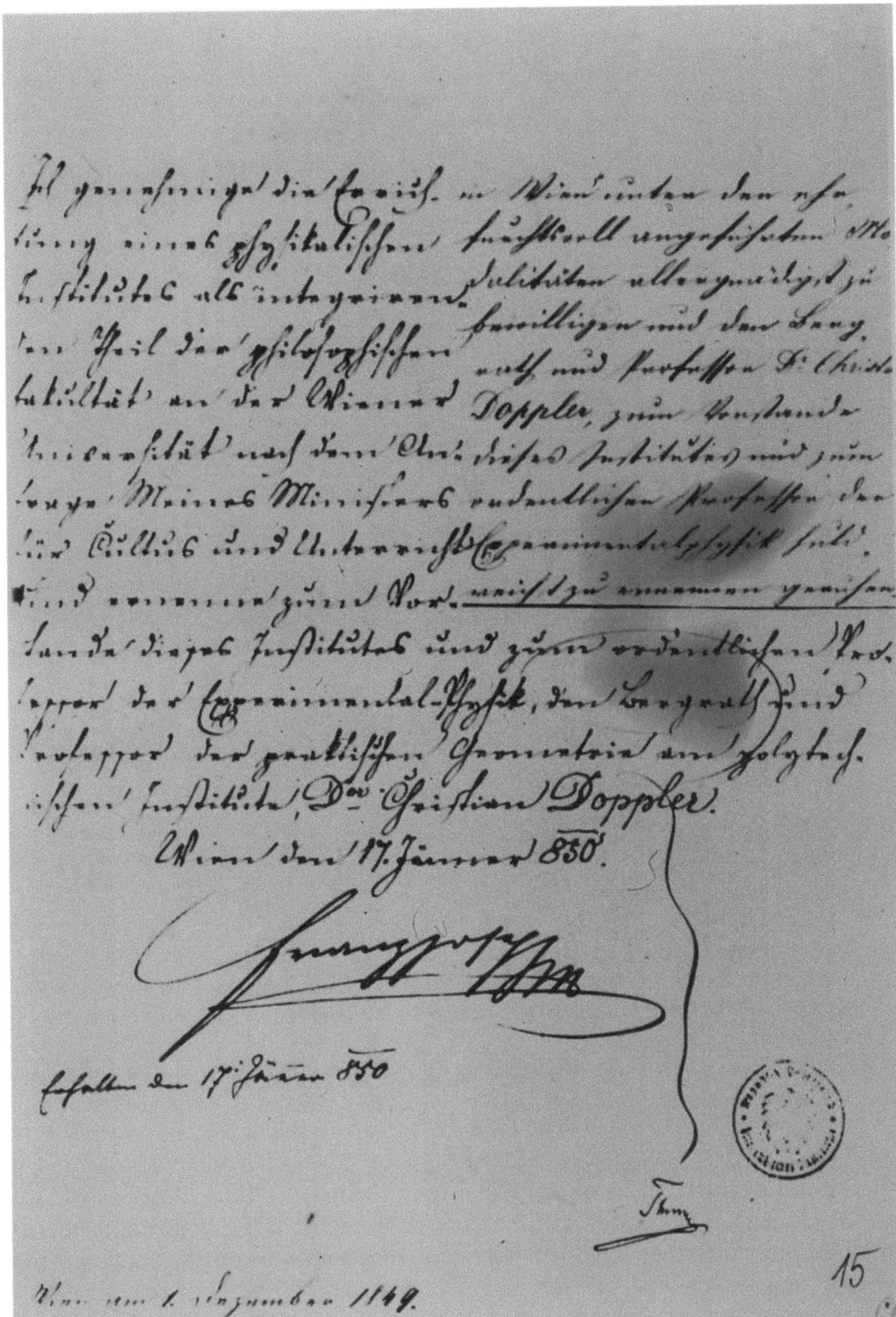
Ich genehmige die Errichtung eines physikalischen Institutes als integrirenden Theil der philosophischen Facultät an der Wiener Universität nach dem Antrage Meines Ministers für Cultus und Unterricht und ernenne zum Vorstande dieses Institutes und zum ordentlichen Professor der Experimental-Physik den Bergrath und Professor der practischen Geometrie am polytechnischen Institute, Dr. Christian Doppler.

in Wien unter den erforderlich angesetzten Modalitäten allergnädigst zu bewilligen und den Bergrath und Professor Dr. Christian Doppler, zum Vorstande dieses Institutes und zum ordentlichen Professor der Experimentalphysik huld-

reichst zu ernennen geruhen.

Wien den 17. Jänner 850.

Franz Joseph

Erhalten den 17. Jänner 850

Thun

Wien am 1. Dezember 1849.

15

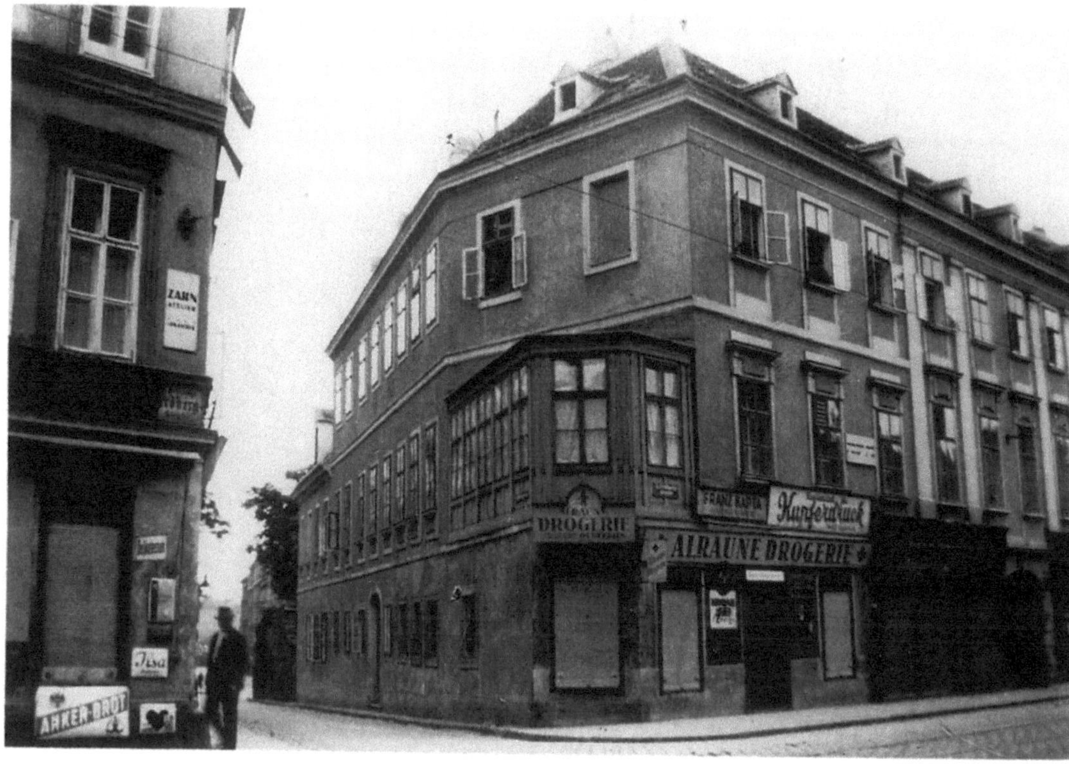

The building in the *Erdbergstrasse* in Vienna which housed Doppler's Institute of Physics. The garden at the rear was used for large scale experiments and Doppler, together with his wife and five small children, occupied the rooftop apartment.

(From the pictorial archives of the Austrian National Library, Vienna)

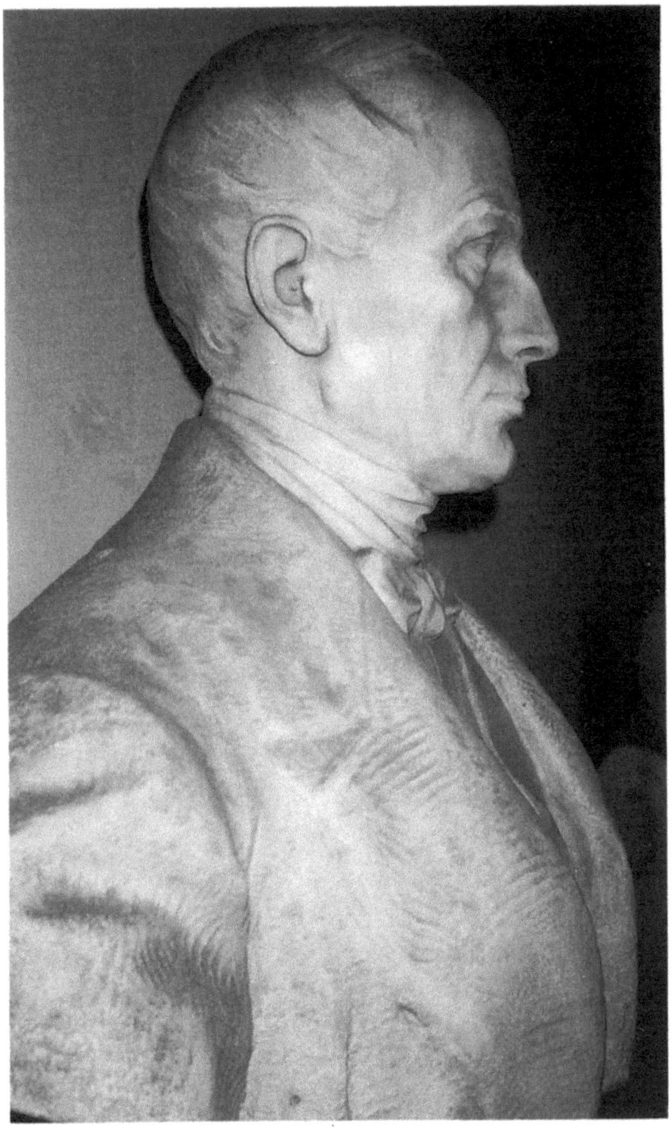

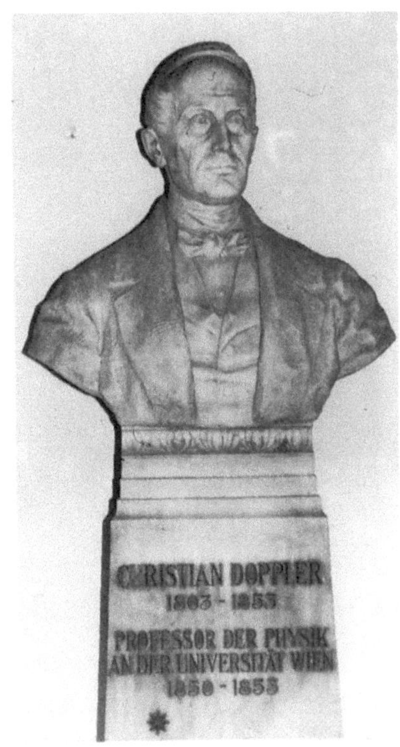

CHRISTIAN DOPPLER
1803 - 1853
PROFESSOR DER PHYSIK
AN DER UNIVERSITÄT WIEN
1850 - 1853

A profile of the bust of Christian Doppler by G. Leiseck, erected in the colonnades of Vienna University in 1901.

(Photographs by the author)

Death in Venice

In my biographical sketch of Doppler published in 1988 I was able to present very little information on the last months of his life in Venice except to establish beyond all doubt, from the entry of death in the records of the municipal archives, the fact that he did die there. In an "epilogue" in this book I raised more questions than I had answered. Although the records of death established that he had died in the parish of *San Giovanni in Bragora* (St. John in the Swamp), I had been unable to locate the house. Neither could I, despite several days spent searching through the beautiful cemetery on the Island of St. Michael, find Doppler's gravestone, nor even the stone tablet that had been erected in his memory by the physicists of Venice following his death in 1853. I incorrectly attributed a completely illegible tablet of deceptively similar design (since shown to be a memorial to the *Famiglia Marseille*) as being the remains of the Doppler memorial, and raised strong doubts as to whether Doppler was actually buried in Venice. "These questions remain unanswered", I wrote then, "and the truth is — whether in Venice or elsewhere — we do not know where Christian Doppler's grave is. The author has not yet given up the search."

These doubts — and similar uncertainties concerning Doppler's final resting place that I had expressed in a medical publication in 1986 (34) — prompted others into investigating this apparent mystery. The neurologists at the University Hospital in Venice worked together with a journalist to research the last days of Doppler in Venice and from them we have much information about his death and burial on the *Isola San Michele* (10, 88). But it is the Viennese physicist-writer, Dr. Peter Schuster, to whom we must give credit for first unearthing further details of the Doppler memorial and the location of the house in which he died (78). From these and other sources, we now have a number of documents concerning the last five months of Doppler's life, his death and burial on the *Isola San Michele* — but still no firm evidence concerning the exact site of his grave. As have others before him (17, 43, 44), Schuster commits the error of referring to the memorial stone as Doppler's grave. However reluctantly, I must agree with Joachim Aubert who in 1975 wrote of Doppler: "*Grab nicht mehr nachweisbar*" (Grave no longer to be located) (3).

When Doppler arrived in Venice during November 1852, he took lodgings in the house number 3758 which overlooks the *Campiello del Piovan* with the background of the 7th century parish church of *San Giovanni in Bragora* in which the musician Antonio Vivaldi had been baptised some 180

years earlier. My Venetian friends told me that this was the courtyard in which the priests from the Church of *San Giovanni in Bragora* would take their walks. From the *Anagrafi* for 1850 in the Venetian Municipal Archives we can establish that this was then in possession of the Tilling family, of whom Wilhelm had been the Austrian Consul-General to the Province of Venice and it was perhaps through this connection that Doppler had arranged to stay there and to be attended by Dr. Pitans who would visit him regularly. It has been suggested that their young housemaid, Antonia Pierobon, helped to attend the sick man (88). The mild climate and sea air of Venice — considered to be rich in iodine salts — made it a popular destination for those seeking palliation for pulmonary tuberculosis in those days.

We really have no way of knowing how Christian Doppler spent those last five months of his life in Venice. Was he was able to look around that beautiful city, or was he confined to his lodgings — or even to his bed? Perhaps he experienced all three states as his health progressively deteriorated and he neared his end. One thing is apparent: true to his nature, Christian Doppler worked! This is clear from a number of handwritten manuscripts that have recently come to light.

Among them are three scientific works, one of which is in a completed form. These were apparently found in Doppler's lodgings on his death and were handed over to his son Adolf. They were perhaps among the manuscripts sent by him to the astronomer Professor Egon von Oppolzer in 1904, together with the family portrait shown on page 46. After giving advice on where to have the daguerreotype restored, von Oppolzer wrote from his home in Innsbruck: "I would advise you to donate the manuscripts to a public institute and would recommend Salzburg as the most suitable place." Well, these (and the daguerreotype) are now in Salzburg — in the safe keeping of the Christian Doppler Foundation — but they have only recently arrived, and by a very circuitous route!

Doppler's son Adolf did not heed the advice of Professor Oppolzer, but retained these manuscripts within the Doppler family, firstly to the son of his brother Hermann — also called Adolf Doppler, from whom we have the many biographical notes — and then to his sister Hermine, who did not marry. Hermine Doppler was, as Doppler's great granddaughter Dorothea Merstallinger told me, a somewhat strange lady who cut herself off from the rest of the Doppler relatives, so it was only some time after the event that they learned of her death in Vienna in 1975 at the age of 83. The many valuable items of her grandfather's work, which it was planned to bequeath

to the Austrian Academy of Sciences, were not to be found. There was a police enquiry from which it emerged that these valuable documents had been sold to a secondhand dealer and that some had been purchased by a retired professor, Dr. Josef Richling (79). Following considerable correspondence, I met with Dr. Richling in Vienna in 1987 to discuss with him the purchase of this Doppler memorabilia for the Christian Doppler Foundation which was then in planning. A further meeting was arranged at which he promised to show me some of these possessions and others of which he knew the whereabouts. He died suddenly before this meeting could take place, and it was not until early 1990 that Professor Gunther Ladurner, Vice President of the Foundation in Salzburg, was able to locate and secure these priceless documents.

The first of seven pages of a completed work is shown on page 71. It is entitled: "On the possibility of determining the number and the absolute distance of the atoms, as well as their reciprocal force of attraction, firstly with various simple solid bodies." A somewhat abridged version of this was published by the Austrian Academy of Sciences in 1953 to celebrate the 150th anniversary of Doppler's birthday and the 100th anniversary of his death (28). The manuscript was made available by Doppler's grandson Adolf, in whose possession it was at that time, and it is noted in the Yearbook of the Academy for 1953 that "It is from the year of the death of the discoverer of the Doppler principle". Certainly someone has pencilled on the top lefthand corner of the manuscript "Venice, January 1853" — the handwriting is not Doppler's.

Peter Schuster, on the other hand, dates this work from Doppler's time in Prague and points out (42) that at a meeting of the Royal Bohemian Society of Sciences held there on 20th May 1846 it is minuted: "Doppler spoke in an extemporaneous lecture on the possibility of determining by experimental means the absolute conditions as well as the absolute number of the atoms that constitute a solid body." But this was an impromptu lecture, perhaps made without notes, and it is in keeping with Doppler's character that when he went to Venice, probably realising that he did not have much longer to live, he used his last days to document those ideas to which he had given much thought — surely also the subject of discussion and even unscripted lectures — but which he had not yet brought to paper. A further handwritten document is entitled: "Thoughts on the possibility of finding the absolute distance as well as the absolute number of the molecules contained in a solid body" which is a rough draft that could have formed the basis for the finished article (page 71). "Remarks on the theory of atoms" is the title on another handwritten document of three pages,

with illustrations, indicating that Doppler had given considerable and precocious thought to this subject on which he never published during his lifetime.

As the Venetian winter of 1852—1853 came to a close, so did the life of Christian Doppler. We learn from the handwritten entry of his wife Mathilde (page 72), that she left her children, probably in the care of her fifteen year-old daughter, to arrive in Venice on 12th March 1853. Five days later, less than four months after his 49th birthday, he was to die in the early hours of the morning, "painlessly and quietly in the arms of his devoted wife" (80) in the small room overlooking the courtyard where the priests took their daily stroll.

His death is recorded in the Municipal Archives and also in the Parish Register of *San Giovanni in Bragora*, where the number of the house is noted (page 73). This entry ends with the abbreviation "Cap." which is an ecclesiastical term "Capitolo", meaning a grand funeral to be attended by all the priests of the parish. This was held on the following day at 2 p. m. in the Church of *San Giovanni in Bragora* and a report in the *Gazzetta Uffiziale di Venezia* for March notes many of the academic and civil dignitaries that attended.

Doppler's wife Mathilde left Venice on 20th March to return to her five young children in Vienna (page 72).

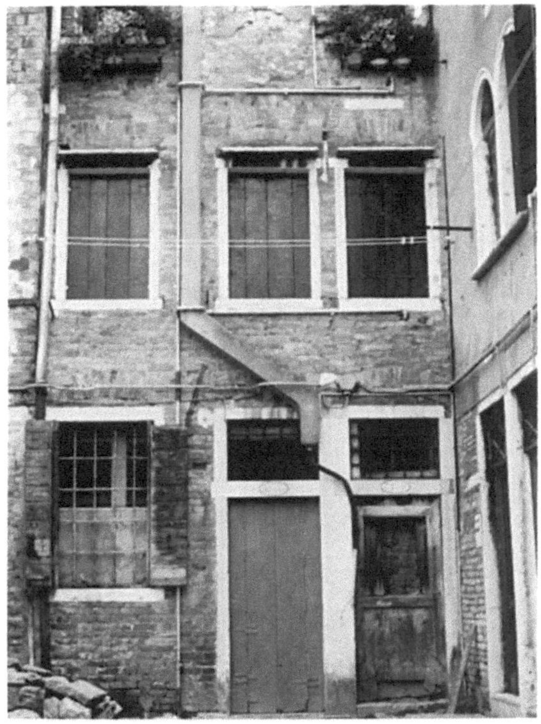

House No: 3758 on the *Campiello del Piovan* in Venice in which Christian Doppler died in the early morning of 17th March 1853.

(Photograph by the author)

The first pages of a rough draft (left) and the completed work entitled "On the possibility of determining the number and the absolute distance of the atoms, as well as their reciprocal force of attraction, firstly with various simple solid bodies". This is thought to have been made by Doppler in Venice in January 1852, three months before his death.

(Original manuscripts kindly donated to the Christian Doppler Foundation in Salzburg by its Vice President, Professor Gunther Ladurner)

Gedanken über die Möglichkeit, die absoluten Abstände sowohl wie die absolute Anzahl der einen festen Körper ~~bildenden~~ constituirenden einzelnen Moleküle zu finden.

Es liegt ohne Zweifel ein sehr großer [illegible] Reiz darin, Umschau zu halten und darüber nachzuforschen, ob es nicht denn [illegible] wird, das Innere der Natur [illegible] mehr zu erschließen, um das Wesen der verschiedenen Erscheinungen [illegible] den Schleier [illegible] haben, doch wenig [illegible] lüften, und der Natur [illegible] ihr geheimes Wirken [illegible].

Ein ungemein wichtiger Schritt wäre in dieser Beziehung nach vorwärts [illegible], wenn es uns gelänge, sowohl die absoluten Abstände als auch die absolute Anzahl derjenigen Moleküle zu bestimmen, aus denen wir uns die verschiedenen Körper zusammengesetzt vorstellen müssen. ~~[illegible]~~ Bisher ist in dieser Beziehung so viel mir bekannt, noch nichts geschehen, ja nicht einmal eine Ahnung [illegible] ~~[illegible]~~ [illegible] in der Wissenschaft geltend gemacht, und man hegt diesfalls nur die allerdings richtige Ansicht, dass jene Abstände jedenfalls ganz ungeheuer klein, ~~[illegible]~~ die Anzahl der Moleküle daher als Folge dessen unendlich groß sein müssen.

Nicht also eine Beantwortung jener Fragen, eine vollständige Lösung der ~~[illegible]~~ angeregten Aufgabe verspreche ich hier zu geben, — sondern nur durch Hinweisung auf [illegible] Weg, die Aussicht zu eröffnen beabsichtige ich durch die gegenwärtige Mittheilung. —

Das Gesetz nach welchem die Molekularanziehung mit der Anziehung [illegible] im Allgemeinen, so wie ~~[illegible]~~ [illegible] oder specielle Verhältnisse für die einzelnen starren und flüssigen Körper kennt man noch nicht, man ~~[illegible]~~ [illegible] hat angenommen, dass die Molekularkraft [illegible] in einem [illegible] weit rascheren Verhältnisse abnehmen als das Quadrat der [illegible] — [illegible] die Abstände [illegible] sich immer [illegible] der [illegible] an, [illegible] als die Abnahme einer Länge gelten, während man die anderen [illegible] Ursachen der Äußerungen der Attraction oder Molekularanziehung [illegible], wobei die [illegible] als [illegible] wurde; so begreift man auch von allen die [illegible] zu bestimmen [illegible] Gradienten [illegible] [illegible] die beiden andern [illegible] in der Formel $y = \frac{c t}{x^n \times [illegible]}$ begriffen.

Newton hält gleichfalls dafür dass in $\frac{ct}{x^n}$ als Ausdruck für die ~~[illegible]~~ Größe der Attraction $n > 2$ sein [illegible] [illegible] pag 26 [illegible]

[illegible]

1.

Ueber die Möglichkeit
die Anzahl* und den absoluten Abstand der Körperatome,
so wie das Maß der wechselseitigen
Anziehungskräfte
zwischen beiden verschiedenen einfachen festen Körpern
zu bestimmen.
von
Dr. Christian Doppler

Venedig
Jänner
1853.

§1. [illegible]

§2 [illegible]

*. Anmerkung. [illegible]

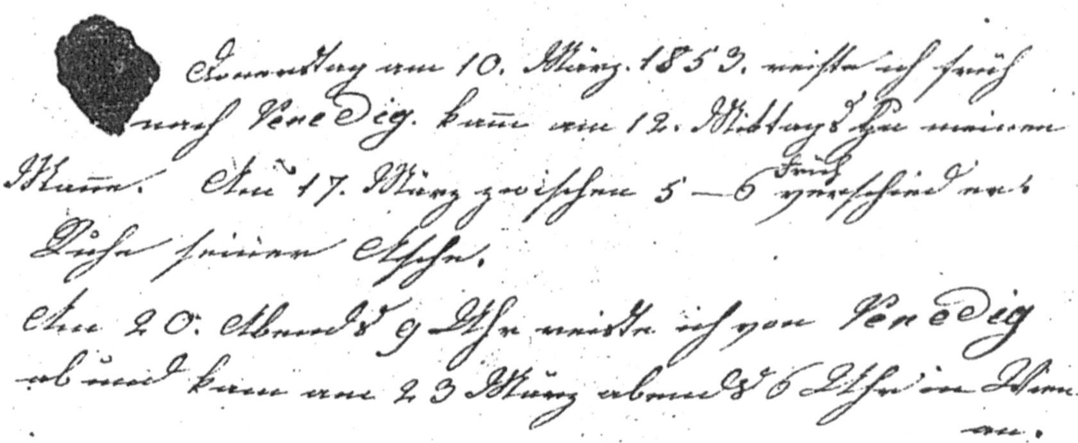
Donnerstag am 10. März 1853. reiste ich früh
nach Venedig. kam am 12. Mittags zu meinem
Mann. Am 17. März zwischen 5–6 früh verschied mein
[illegible]
Am 20. Abends 9 Uhr reiste ich von Venedig
ab und kam am 23 März abends 6 Uhr in Wien
an.

A handwritten note by Doppler's wife, Mathilde, apparently taken from a diary or similar notebook. It bears the imprint of her signet ring or seal in wax on left-hand corner and reads:

Thursday, 10th March 1853, I travelled early from Vienna and came on the 12th at midday to my husband. On 17th March between 5 and 6 in the morning he departed this life. May he rest in peace. On the 20th at 9 in the evening I travelled from Venice and arrived on 23rd March at 6 in the evening in Vienna.

(Original kindly donated to the Christian Doppler Foundation in Salzburg by Frau Dorothea Merstallinger, the great granddaughter of Christian Doppler)

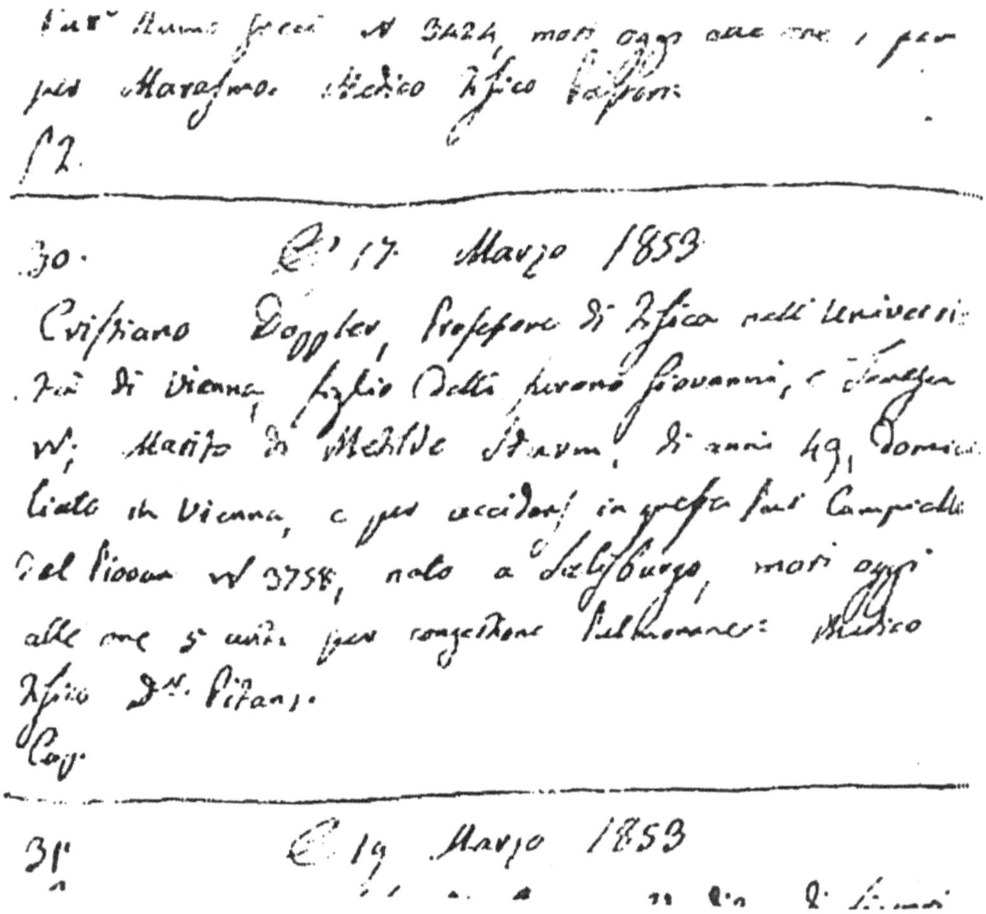

30. Li 17 Marzo 1853
Cristiano Doppler, Professore di Fisica nell'Universi-
tà di Vienna, figlio delli furono Giovanni, e Teresa
W; Marito di Mathilde Sturm, di anni 49, Domici-
liato in Vienna, e per accidente in questa Par. Campiello
del Piovan N. 3758, nato a Salisburgo, morì oggi
alle ore 5 ant. per congestione Polmonare: Medico
Fisico Dr. Pitans.
Cap.

31. Li 19 Marzo 1853

Entry of Doppler's death in the parish records of *San Giovanni in Bragora.* It reads:

17th March 1853
Christian Doppler, Professor of Physics at the University of Vienna, son of Johann and Teresa W; married to Mathilda Sturm, aged 49, domiciled in Vienna and by chance in this Parish. Campiello del Piovan no: 3758, born in Salzburg, died today at 5 a. m. from pulmonary congestion: Medical attendant Dr. Pitans.
Cap.

(Registro dei Morti n. XXVI — Parrocchia di San Giovanni in Bragora, Venezia)

Mathilde Doppler, geborne Sturm, gibt in ihrem und im Namen ihrer minderjährigen Kinder: Mathilde, Ludwig, Adolf, Bertha und Hermann, die tief betrübende Nachricht von dem Hinscheiden ihres Gemahls, resp. Vaters, des Herrn

Christian Doppler,

Dr. der Philosophie, ordentl. Professor der Physik an der k. k. Universität zu Wien, emerit. k. k. Bergrath, ordentl. Mitglied der k. k. Akademie der Wissenschaften zu Wien, Prag und mehrerer anderen gelehrten Gesellschaften.

Er entschlief im 50. Jahre seines Alters nach längerem Leiden am 17. März 1853 zu Venedig selig in dem Herrn.

Die heil. Seelenmessen werden in verschiedenen Kirchen gelesen.

The formal announcement of Doppler's death. It reads:

Mathilde Doppler, née Sturm, announces also in the names of her young children: Mathilde, Ludwig, Adolf, Bertha and Hermann, the deeply distressing news of the passing away of their husband and father
Christian Doppler
Doctor of Philosophy, Professor of Physics at the Imperial University of Vienna, Imperial *Bergrath emeritus*, Member of the Imperial Academy of Science in Vienna, Prague and many other learned societies.

He fell asleep in the 50th year of his life, after a long suffering on 17th March 1853 in Venice, blessed in the Lord.

The Holy Requiem will be held in various churches.

(Copy kindly provided by Dorothea Merstallinger, Christian Doppler's great granddaughter)

Epilogue

Following Doppler's death a formally printed and eloquent message of condolence to the Faculty of Philosophy of the Imperial University in Vienna was sent out by Professor Francesco Zantedeschi on behalf of the scientists of Venice and at the end of the long Venetian summer of 1853 a memorial was erected by them, with permission from the city council, in the arcades of the cemetery on the *Isola San Michele* (page 76). The eulogy of Professor Bernardo Zambra was published in the *Gazzetta Uffiziale di Venezia* of 15th September 1853.

On March 18th 1990 the *Gazzettino di Venezia* carried another report about a similar ceremony at the restored Doppler memorial. On the previous day, the 137th anniversary of the death of the Salzburg physicist, the Governor of the State of Salzburg and the Mayor of Venice, together with the President of the Christian Doppler Foundation, laid wreaths during a short ceremony at the memorial. Dignitaries from Salzburg and Venice were present, as well as descendants of Christian Doppler. This solemn act in remembrance of the modest and industrious family man had been preceded by the unveiling of a commemorative tablet on the front side of the house in which he had died.

Provided by the Christian Doppler Foundation, the tablet is made of marble from the quarries of the *Untersberg* near Salzburg, which was formerly worked by the Doppler Family, and it was engraved at the old Doppler stonemasonry in *Himmelreich*. It reads*:

In questa casa
il 17. Marzo 1853 mori
Il grande
fisico e matematico austriaco
CHRISTIAN DOPPLER
che scopri
l'EFFETO DOPPLER

n. Salisburgo, 29. Novembre 1803
m. Venezia 17. Marzo 1853

* *In this house on 17th March 1853 died the great Austrian physicist and mathematician, Christian Doppler, discoverer of the Doppler effect. Born Salzburg 29th November 1803. Died Venice 17th March 1853.*

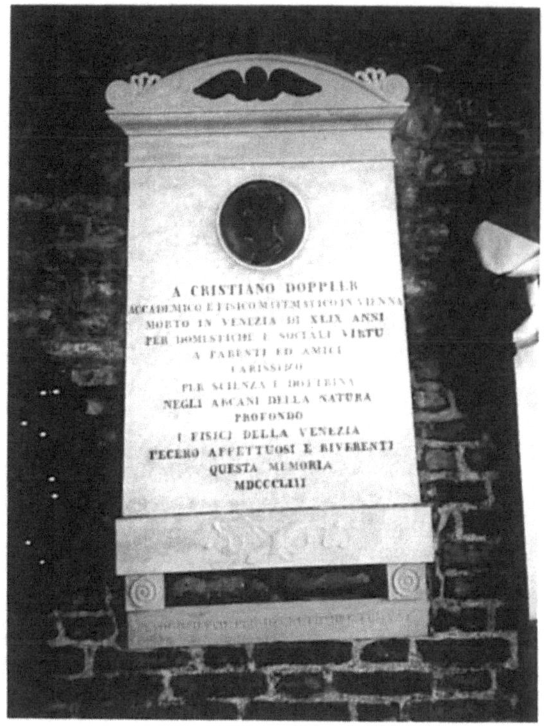

The restored memorial to Doppler in the arcades of the Venetian cemetery on the *Isola San Michele.* It reads:

TO CHRISTIAN DOPPLER
ACADEMICIAN AND MATHEMATICAL PHYSICIST IN VIENNA
DIED IN VENICE AGED 49 YEARS.
THROUGH DOMESTIC AND SOCIAL VIRTUE
MUCH LOVED BY RELATIVES AND FRIENDS.
THROUGH SCIENCE AND LEARNING
PENETRATED DEEP INTO THE SECRETS OF NATURE.
THE PHYSICISTS OF VENICE
AFFECTIONATELY AND REVERENTLY
DEDICATE
THIS MEMORIAL
1853
Location donated by resolution of the council

References

1. Anderlik, G. (1972) Christian Doppler, Auch ein Wegbereiter in der Astronautik. In: In Salzburg geboren. Salzburger Nachrichten Verlags GmbH, Salzburg, pp 156—160

2. Andrade, E. N. da C. (1959) Doppler and the Doppler Effect. Endeavour **18**: 14—19

3. Aubert, J. (1975) Handbuch der Grabstätten berühmter Deutscher, Österreicher und Schweizer. Deutscher Kunstverlag,.München Berlin, p 189

4. Bolzano, B. (1837) Letter to the Royal Bohemian Society of Sciences, Prague, dated 25. 9. 1837. Archives of the Czechoslovakian Academy of Sciences

5. Bolzano, B. (1843) Ein Paar Bemerkungen über die neue Theorie in Herrn Professor Ch. Doppler's Schrift: „Über das farbige Licht der Doppelsterne und einiger anderer Gestirne des Himmels." Pogg. Annal. der Physik und Chemie **60**: 83

6. Bolzano, B. (1847) Christian Doppler's neueste Leistungen auf dem Gebiet der physikalischen Apparatenlehre, Akustik, Optik und optischen Astronomie. Pogg. Annal. der Physik und Chemie, **72**: 530—555

7. Bradley, J. (1729) An account of a new discovered motion of the fixed stars. Phil. Trans. Roy. Soc. (London) **35**: 637—661

8. Buberl, P., F. Martin (1915) Grossgmain. Sonderabdruck aus der österreichischen Kunsttopographie, Band XI, Wien

9. Buys Ballot, C. H. D. (1845) Akustische Versuche auf der Niederländischen Eisenbahn nebst gelegentlichen Bemerkungen zur Theorie des Hrn. Prof. Doppler. Pogg. Annal. der Physik und Chemie **66**, 321—351

10. Campioni, A., R. Vianello (1989) History of Neurology: contribution to Doppler biography. Ital. J. Neurol. Sci. **10**: 527—528

11. Czihak, G. (1984) Johann Gregor Mendel [1822—1884]. Dokumentierte Biographie und Katalog zur Gedächtnisausstellung anläßlich des hundertsten Todestags. Salzburg

12. Dick, A. (1984) Gründung und Ausstattung des k. k. physikalischen Institutes der Universität Wien. Lecture presented at the Gregor Mendel Symposium, Vienna, 2. 2. 1984

13. Doppler, A. (1943) Manuscript in the Archives of the Technical University, Vienna

14. Doppler, A. (1953) Christian Doppler. Natur und Technik **7**: 68—69

15. Doppler, C. (1832) Beitrag zu den Paralleltheorien. Wien Polytechn. Jahrb. **17**

16. Doppler, C. (1834) Über die wahrscheinliche Ursache der Elecktricitäts-Erregung durch Berührung. Wien Polytechn. Jahrb. **18**

17. Doppler, C. (1842) Über das farbige Licht der Doppelsterne und einiger anderer Gestirne des Himmels. Abhandl. königl. böhm. Gesellsch. d. Wiss. **2**: 465—482

18. Doppler, C. (1843) Arithmetik und Algebra mit besonderer Rücksicht auf die Bedürfnisse der verschiedenen Wissenschaften und des praktischen Lebens, mit einem Anhange von 450 Aufgaben und Beispielen. Borrosch & André, Prague (2nd Edition, Braumüller, Wien 1851)

19. Doppler, C. (1844) Beleuchtung und Wiederbelegung der von Dr. Maedler in Dorpat gegen die Theorie des farbigen Lichtes der Doppelsterne gemachten Einwendungen und Bedenken. Österr. Blätter f. Lit. u. Kunst **15**

20. Doppler, C. (1846) Bemerkungen zu meiner Theorie des farbigen Lichtes der Doppelsterne etc., mit vorzüglicher Rücksicht auf die von Herrn Dr. Ballot zu Utrecht dagegen erhobenen Bedenken. Pog. Ann. **68**: 1—35

21. Doppler, C. (1849) Über eine noch unbenützte Quelle magnetischer Declinationsbeobachtungen. Sitzungsber. d. Kaiserl. Akad. d. Wiss. (Wien) **2**: 249

22. Doppler, C. (1849) Über eine Reihe markscheiderischer Declinationsbeobachtungen aus der Zeit 1735—1736. Sitzungsber. d. Kaiserl. Akad. d. Wiss. (Wien) **3**: 1—4

23. Doppler, C. (1850) Bemerkungen und Anträge, die magnetischen Beobachtungsdaten aus Joachimsthal, Freiburg etc. betreffend. Sitzungsber. d. Kaiserl. Akad. d. Wiss. (Wien) **4**: 336

24. Doppler, C. (1851) Über die Anwendung der Syrene und des akustischen Flugrädchens zur Bestimmung des Spannungsgrades der Wasserdämpfe und der comprimierten Luft. Sitzungsber. d. Kaiserl. Akad. d. Wiss. (Wien) **6**: 206—214

25. Doppler, C. (1851) Letter to the Imperial Ministry of Culture and Education dated 16. 4. 1851 concerning the draft contract for the house No. 104 in the Hauptstrasse in Erdberg. Austrian National Archives, General Administrative Archives No. 4036/851

26. Doppler, C. (1852) Bemerkungen zu dem Aufsatze: „Über ein allgemeines Princip der Undulationslehre: Gesetz der Erhaltung der Schwingungsdauer." Sitzungsber. d. Kaiserl. Akad. d. Wiss. (Wien) **8**: 587—593

27. Doppler, C. (1852) Bemerkungen über die von Herrn Prof. Petzval gegen die Richtigkeit meiner Theorie vorgebrachten Einwendungen. Sitzungsber. d. Kaiserl. Akad. d. Wiss. (Wien) **9**: 217—225

28. Doppler, C. (1852?) Über die Möglichkeit, die Anzahl und den absoluten Abstand der Körperatome sowie das Maß ihrer wechselseitigen Anziehungsstärke zunächst bei den

verschiedenen einfachen festen Körpern zu bestimmen. In: Jahrb. d. österr. Akad. d. Wiss. (Wien) 1953 pp 498—514

29. Doppler, Theresia (1830) Statement to the Civil Court in Salzburg, 8. 2. 1830. Salzburg State Archives

30. Dorland, W. A. (1936) The American Illustrated Medical Dictionary. W. B. Saunders Company, Philadelphia London, p 420

31. Eden, A. (1984) Cerebrovascular Doppler Sonography: Recent Advances and Developments. Lecture as Visiting Professor, Health Sciences Center, University of Texas at Dallas

32. Eden, A. (1985) An early history of Doppler. Proc. Symp. Ultrasound Diag. Cerebrovasc. Dis. IAPM, Seattle

33. Eden, A. (1985) Johann Christian Doppler? Ultrasound Med. Biol. **11**: 537—539

34. Eden, A. (1986) The beginnings of Doppler. In: Transcranial Doppler Sonography (Ed.: R. Aaslid) Springer-Verlag, Wien New York, pp 1—9

35. Eden, A. (1988) Johann Christian Doppler? Oder Christian Andreas Doppler? Dtsch. Med. Wochenschr. **113**: 158—159

36. Eden, A. (1988) Christian Doppler: Thinker and Benefactor. The Christian Doppler Institute for Medical Science and Technology, Salzburg

37. Eden, A. (1990) The Doppler effect: general considerations. Diagn. Interv. Radiol. **2**: 67

38. Ettingshausen, A. von (1852) Weitere Bemerkungen zu dem Vortrag des Herrn Prof. Petzval vom 15. 1. 1852. Sitzungsber. d. Kaiserl. Akad. d. Wiss. (Wien) **9**: 226—229

39. Folta, J. (1981) The Life and Scientific Endeavour of Bernard Bolzano. In: Bolzano and the Foundations of Mathematical Analysis (Ed.: V. Jarník) Society of Czechoslovakian Mathematicians and Physicists, Prague

40. Franceschi, V., D. Vadrot (1989) The Doppler Effect: General Considerations. Diag. Interv. Radiol. **1**: 75—77

41. Gassauer, T. (1950) Die wissenschaftliche Kontroverse zwischen Petzval und Doppler. Dissertation for the degree of Doctor of Philosophy at the University of Vienna

42. Grössing, H., P. Schuster (1992) Christian Doppler, 1803—1853. Böhlau Verlag, Vienna (in press)

43. Haas, K. (1904) Christian Doppler und seine Entdeckungen. Vierteljahresber. d. Wiener Vereines zur Förderung d. Physik u. chem. Unterrichtes (Wien) 9—22

44. Hach, W. (1987) Das Lebensbild des Johann Christian Doppler. Dtsch. Med. Wochenschr. **112**: 1314—1317

45. Hach, W. (1988) Johann Christian Doppler? Oder Christian Andreas Doppler? Dtsch. Med. Wochenschr. **113**: 158—159

46. Hannsmann, L. (1965) Johann Christian Doppler v Banskej Štiavnici. Zprávy Společnosti pro dejiny věd a techniky **1**: 61—62

47. Havránek, J. (1981) František Palacky a Univerzita Karlova. Acta Universitatis Carolinae Pragensis **XXI**: 67—81

48. Hübner, L. (1796) Beschreibung des Erzstiftes und Reichsfürstentumes Salzburg, Vol. 1, p 138

49. Herchel, J. F. W. (1800) Experiments on the Refrangibility of the Invisible Rays of the Sun. Phil. Trans. Royal Soc. (London) **90**: 284—292

50. Jäger, G. (1926) Christian Doppler. In: Neue österreichische Biographie. Amalthea-Verlag, Wien, pp 72—81

51. Jelinek, K. (1856) Das ständ.-polytechnische Institut zu Prag. Haase, Prag

52. Jonkmann, E. J. (1980) Doppler research in the nineteenth century. Ultrasound Med. Biol. **6**: 1—5

53. Klein, H. (1952) Aus der Baugeschichte des Dopplerhauses. Bastei, Salzburg **3**: 3—5

54. Korinek, R. (1982) Grossgmain in Flachau. Buchhandlung Korinek, Grossgmain, pp 22—23

55. Kral, J. (1939) Christian Doppler: Lebensbild eines großen Salzburgers. Salzburger Volksblatt, 3.—4. 1. 1939

56. Kreil, K. (1853) Letters dated (a) 27. 4. 1853 and (b) 12. 5. 1853 to Prof. Anton Schrötter, Secretary General of the Imperial Academy of Sciences. Archives of the Austrian Academy of Sciences, Vienna

57. Kunz, E. (1893) Über Christian Doppler. Mitteilungen d. Gesellsch. f. Salzburger Landeskunde **33**: 201—206

58. Kunz, E. (1903) Christian Doppler. Zur Feier seines hundertsten Geburtstages. Vortrag gehalten in der Gesellschaft für Salzburger Landeskunde am 28. November 1903

59. Lorentz, H. A. (1907) Abhandlungen von Christian Doppler. Verlag Wilhelm Engelman, Leipzig

60. Mache, H. (1937) Österreichs große Physiker und ihre Spitzenleistungen. JuV Verlag, Wien, pp 6—7

61. New Century Cyclopedia of Names (1955) p 1313

62. O'Donnell, K. P., D. F. Powers, J. McCarthy (1970) Johnny, we hardly knew ye. Little, Brown and Company, Boston Toronto, pp 30—31

63. Oppolzer, E. von (1901) Festrede bei Enthüllung des Doppler-Denkmales im Arkadenhof der k. k. Universität zu Wien. Neue Freie Presse, Wien, 7. November 1901

64. Ortner, G. (1951) Christian Doppler: Ein Wegbereiter für Physik und Astronomie. In: Österreichische Naturforscher und Techniker. Verlag der Gesellschaft für Natur und Technik, Wien

65. Parkinson, W. D. (1983) An Introduction to Geomagnetism, Edinburgh

66. Petráň, J. (1988) Das Karolinium. Karlsuniversität Prag, p 45

67. Petzval, J. (1853) Über ein allgemeines Princip der Undulationslehre: Gesetz der Erhaltung der Schwingungsdauer. Sitzungsber. d. Kaiserl. Akad. d. Wiss. (Wien) **8:** 134

68. Petzval, J. (1852) Über die Unkömmlichkeiten gewisser populärer Anschauungsweisen in der Undulationstheorie und ihre Unfähigkeit das Prinzip der Erhaltung der Schwingungsdauer zu ersetzen. Sitzungsber. d. Kaiserl. Akad. d. Wiss. (Wien) **8:** 384

69. Pöss, O. (1991) Von einer wenig bekannten Aktivität Christian Dopplers. IV. Conference on the History of Physics, Dresden

70. Poscke, F. (1896) Johann Christian Doppler und das Dopplersche Prinzip. Zeitschr. f. d. physik. u. chem. Unterricht. Springer, Berlin, 248—249

71. Quittner, V. (1904) Christian Doppler. Prometheus **15:** 113—116

72. Reischel, B. (1990) Personal communication

73. Ritter, J. W. (1801) Ausfindung nicht sichtbarer Sonnenstrahlen außerhalb des Farbenspectrums an die Seite des Violetts. Wiederholung der Rouppachen Versuche mit Kohle. Annalen der Physik 7: 525

74. Royal Bohemian Society of Sciences (1842—1843). Minutes of the Meetings of (a) 25. 5. 1842, (b) 5. 11. 1843, (c) 3. 12. 1843 and (d) 31. 12. 1843. Archives of the Czechoslovakian Academy of Sciences, Prague

75. Royal Bohemiam Society of Sciences (1844). Letter dated 15th January 1844 to Christian Doppler. Archives of the Czechoslovakian Academy of Sciences, Prague

76. Russell, J. S. (1848) On certain effects produced on sound by the rapid motion of the observer. Brit. Assn. Rep. **18:** 37

77. Scheiner, J. (1896) Johann Christian Doppler und das nach ihm benannte Prinzip. Himmel und Erde **8:** 260—271

78. Schuster, P. (1989) Eine Rose für Christian Doppler. Falter (Wien) **15:** 11—15

79. Schuster, P. (1989) Die Enthüllung des Dopplerportraits. Falter (Wien) **30:** 9

80. Schrötter, A. (1854) Bericht des G. Secretärs. Almanach d. Kaiserl. Akad. d. Wiss. (Wien) 112—120

81. St. Andrä in Salzburg (1986) Christliche Kunststätten Österreichs Nr. 148. Verlag St. Peter, Salzburg

82. Stedman's Medical Dictionary (1953) Williams & Wilkins, Baltimore, p 398

83. Steinitz, W. (1971) Salzburg Kunst- und Reiseführer. Residenz Verlag, Salzburg

84. Štoll, I. (1991) Mach and the Doppler Effect. In: Ernst Mach and the development of Physics (Eds.: V. Prosser, J. Folta) Charles University, Prague, pp 285—293

85. Studnička, F. J. (1903) Vorwort zu „Über das farbige Licht der Doppelsterne" von Christian Doppler zur Feier seines hundertsten Geburtstages. Verlag der königl. böhm. Gesellschaft der Wissenschaften, Prag

86. Thieme-Becker (1782) Wiener Zeitung **9:** 406

87. Toole, J. F. (1990) Cerebrovascular Disorders (4th Edition, Raven Press, New York) p vii

88. Vianello, R. (1989) Il sogiorno veneziani di Christiano Doppler. Ateneo Veneto, Venezia

89. White, D. N. (1982) Johann Christian Doppler and his Effect. Ultrasound Med. Biol. **8:** 583—591

90. Woodruff, A. E. (1971) Dictionary of Scientific Biography (Ed.: C. C. Gillespie) Vol. IV, New York, pp 167—169

91. Wurzbach, C. von (1858) In: Biographisches Lexicon des Kaiserthums Oesterreich **3:** 370—372

92. Zillner, F. V. (1885) Geschichte der Stadt Salzburg **1:** 388

The Published Works of Christian Doppler

Both Scheiner (1896) and Haas (1904) put the number of scientific works published by Doppler at 51, whereas his grandson, Adolf Doppler (1953) puts these at "about 56 in number". The following documentation — with titles of the works translated into English — confirms that Adolf Doppler is probably living up to his reputation of tending to exaggerate the achievements of his grandfather. My list of 52 works includes the last work of Doppler, probably written during the last months of his life in 1853, but not published until the 100th anniversary of this event in 1953.

It is perhaps the most complete catalogue of Doppler's works, since those published in the Almanac of the Imperial Academy of Sciences in Vienna in 1851 and 1852 and that of J. C. Poggendorf in 1863 are each deficient of a few works. It is based largely on a list of 48 works, now in the archives of the Austrian Academy of Sciences, made by Doppler himself on 28th December 1850. The 47th item on this list is "Diverse works, largely of critical content, in Hessler's Encyclopedic Journal, the Austrian Pages for Literature and Art, the *Gymnasial* Journal, and many others". It is apparent that Doppler did not consider these as scientific publications, and none has been included here. Second editions are not counted as separate works, neither are papers which reappear in a collected edition under a different title.

His first works appeared in the Yearbook of the Viennese Polytechnic *(Wiener polytechn. Jahrb.)* and Baumgartner's Journal of Physics and Mathematics *(Baumgartner's Zeitschrift für Physik und Mathematik)*. In the early days in Prague he favoured Hessler's Encyclopedic Journal *(Hessler's encyclopädische Zeitschrift)* until becoming an associate member of the Royal Bohemian Society of Sciences in 1840, after which he published largely in the Proceedings of that Society *(Abhandlungen der königl. böhm. Gesellschaft der Wissenschaften)*, mostly with special editions being published by Borrosch & André in Prague. His famous treatise "On the coloured light of the double stars" was the first of these. Following Doppler's return to Vienna early in 1849, almost all his scientific works appeared in the minutes of the mathematical and natural sciences section of the Imperial Academy of Sciences *(Sitzungsbericht d. kaiserl. Akademie d. Wissenschaften)* as well as being published by Braumüller in Vienna and in Poggendorf's Annals.

Opposite:

A letter written from Prague in 1845 by Christian Doppler to a correspondent who had obviously asked for his advice on the publication of a book. During this year Doppler was to publish more scientific works (7) than in any other. Despite its formal style, which was usual in these times, the unknown recipient was certainly a friend of Doppler's. It reads:

Sir,

I have received your welcome letter of 13th June and, since I kinow of no person there who fulfills your requirements, I approached the well-known book and publishing house of Borrosch & André to consult them in this matter. I learned here that by far the most advisable course would be for you to give your work in commission to a Viennese publishing house. These would attend to all the necessary announcements and would distribute the book worldwide. Vienna is for Southern Germany what Leipzig is for the North. I myself have done this with all my literary works and one is spared much bother. The publishers Borrosch — or rather their proprietor — moreover expressed the fear that your project could at the present time be spoiled by the fact that we possess, for Germany itself, a number of excellent recent works of a similar tendency. Our best action, in his opinion, is rather to produce a comprehensive and completely faithful review of the data, specially based on as much firsthand information as possible concerning Austria's problems. Do not let what is stated here prevent you from completing with courage the venture you have already begun, and, among the 40 printing and publishing houses one will certainly be found which will carry out and support your project with full activity. Then no book publisher in Austria can afford to do this more easily than a Viennese, since the sales *in loco* are in any case significant. Also such a publisher, when there are prospects of good sales, should be easily prepared to take over at least part of the printing costs himself, before the completion of the subscription.

With special respect I sign, sir,

Prague, 24th June 1845.

Your devoted servant and friend,
Prof. Christian Doppler

(Reproduced by kind permission of the Museum Carolino Augusteum, Salzburg)

Euer Wohlgeboren!

ich habe Ihr geehrtes Schreiben vom 13ten d. M. richtig erhalten, und da ich Ihnen den Ihren Wünschen entsprechend Folge leisten will, mich an die hierortsbekannte thätige Buch- und Verlagshandlung Borrosch et André gewendet, und hierüber Rücksprache zu nehmen. Ich ersuche Sie daher, da sie sich bereit erklärt [illegible] geneigtest sey, Ihr Werk einer thätigen Wiener Buchhandlung in Commission zu geben. Diese besorgt alle nöthigen Aufträge und versendet es in alle Welt. Wien ist für das südliche Deutschland was Leipzig für das nördliche ist. Ich selbst habe es bei allen meinen litterarischen Arbeiten so gemacht, und ich habe dabei vielen Unannehmlichkeiten überhoben. — Die Buchhandlung Borrosch oder vielmehr der Prinzipal Herr [illegible] äußerte die Befürchtung, auch daß Ihr Unternehmen in gegenwärtiger Zeit durch den Umstand sehr beeinträchtigt werden dürfte, daß nun in der That für das eigentliche Deutschland in neuester Zeit ganz vortreffliche Werke gleichen Inhalts bestehen. Ihr Rath wäre, meinte er, [illegible] möglichst auf Autopsie sich stützende Special-Statistik Österreichs [illegible]. — Möge Sie dies, das hier [illegible] nicht abhalten, Ihr begonnenes Unternehmen mit Muth fortzusetzen, und unter den 40 Verlags- und Commissionshandlungen Wiens wird sich gewiß eine finden, die mit aller Thätigkeit Ihr Unternehmen betreibt und fördert. Denn keine Buchhandlung in Österreich kann dieß leichter auf sich nehmen, wie eine Wiener, da der Absatz in loco jedenfalls schon ein bedeutender ist. Auch dürfte sich eine solche, wenn Aussicht auf Absatz ist, leicht dazu verstehen, die Druckkosten selber wenigstens theilweise auf sich zu nehmen, noch vor zu Stande gekommener Subscription. —

Mit besonderer Achtung zeichne ich

Euer Wohlgeboren

Prag den 24t Juni 1845.

ergebenster Diener

Prof. Christian Doppler

1832

1. *Ein Beitrag zu den Parallelen-Theorien.* (A contribution to the theory of parallels.) *Wiener Polytechn. Jahrb.* **17**

2. *Über die Convergenz einer unendlichen Logarithmenfolge.* (On the convergence of an infinite logarithmic series.) *Ibid.*

3. *Über Kettenwurzeln und deren Convergenz.* (On chain roots and their convergence.) *Ibid.*

1834

4. *Über die wahrscheinliche Ursache der Elecktricitäts-Erregung durch Berührung und der elektrischen Spannung.* (On the probable cause of the creation of electricity through contact and the electrical potential.) *Ibid.* **18**

1837

5. *Über die Durchsichtigkeit der Kometenkerne und die Erscheinung der leuchtenden Puncte im Monde.* (On the transparency of the centre on comets and the appearance of the glowing points in moons.) *Baumgartner's Zeitschrift für Physik und Mathematik* **5**: 193

6. *Über eine merkwürdige Eigenthümlichkeit der electrischen Spannung.* (On a strange property of the electrical potential.) *Ibid.* **8**

7. *Einige Betrachtungen über das Große und das Kleine in der Natur.* (Some considerations on the large and small in nature.) *Ibid.*, Neue Folge **5**: 542

1839

8. *Versuch einer analytischen Behandlung beliebig begrenzter und zusammengesetzter Linien, Flächen und Körper etc.* (An attempt at an analytical treatment of arbitarily defined and composed lines, surfaces, bodies, etc.) Special edition of 12 pages and 3 lithographic tables, Haase & Sons, Prague. (Later [1841] published in the *Abhandlungen der königl. böhm. Gesellschaft der Wissenschaften* **1**)

9. *Bedenken rücksichtlich einer beim Zusammenschlagen zweyer Kieselsteine vorgeblich bemerkten electrischen Erscheinung.* (Thoughts concerning an electrical phenomenon noticed by chance on the collision of two flintstones.) *Poggendorf's Annalen der Physik* **49**: 505

1842

10. *Beschreibung eines Instrumentes (eines Cyclographen), um Kreisbögen von beliebig grossen Radien continuirlich zu verzeichnen.* (Description of an instrument [a cyclograph] for the continuous recording of arcs of any size of radius.) *Hesslers* encyclopädische Zeitschrift **2**: 33

11. *Beschreibung eines neuen Instrumentes zum continuirlichen Verzeichnen der sogenannten Descartes'schen Ovallinien.* (Description of a new instrument for the continuous recording of the so-called Cartesian oval lines.) *Ibid.* **9**: 269

12. *Über das farbige Licht der Doppelsterne und einiger anderer Gestirne des Himmels.* (On the coloured light of the double stars and certain other stars of the heavens.) Borrosch & André, Prague. (Later [1843] published in *Abhandlungen der königl. böhm. Gesellschaft der Wissenschaften* **2**: 465—482)

13. *Ein Beitrag zur Electrizitäts-Erzeugung durch Reibung.* (A contribution to the production of electricity through friction.) *Hessler's encyclopädische Zeitschrift* **16**: 337

14. *Versuch einer Erweiterung der analytischen Geometrie auf Grundlage eines neuen Algorithmus.* (An attempt at the expansion of analytical geometry on the basis of a new algorithm.) *Abhandlungen der königl. böhm. Gesellschaft der Wissenschaften* **2**. (Later [1843] published in a special edition of 22 pages and 9 tables by Borrosch & André, Prague.)

1843

15. *Arithmetik und Algebra mit besonderer Rücksicht auf die Bedürfnisse der verschiedenen Wissenschaften und des praktischen Lebens, mit einem Anhange von 450 Aufgaben und Beispielen.* (Textbook of Arithmetic and Algebra with special reference to the requirements of the various sciences and practical life, with an appendix of 450 problems and examples.) Borrosch & André, Prague. (2nd Edition, Braumüller, Vienna, 1851)

1844

16. *Über einige Verbesserungen in der Construction der Messtische.* (On certain improvements in the construction of the surveyor's table.) *Hessler's encyclopädische Zeitschrift* **19**: 385

17. *Beleuchtung und Wiederlegung der von Dr. Maedler in Dorpat gegen die Theorie des farbigen Lichtes der Doppelsterne gemachten Einwendungen und Bedenken.* (Elucidation and rejection of the reservations and objections of Dr. Maedler of Dorpat against the theory of the coloured light of the double stars.) *Österreichischen Blättern für Literatur und Kunst* **15**

18. *Über eine alle bisherigen Metallgemische an Reflexionsvermögen übertreffende und daher zu optischen Zwecken vorzüglich geeignete Legirung.* (On an alloy that exceeds the reflective capacity of all previous metallic mixtures and is therefore eminently suitable for optical purposes.) *Hessler's encyclopädische Zeitschrift* **19:** 389

1845

19. *Allgemeiner und höchst einfacher Beweis des Satzes, dass dieselben Factoren in beliebiger Ordnung multiplicirt stets dasselbe Product geben.* (A general and highly simple proof of the tenet that the same factors multiplied in random order always give the same product.) *Abhandlungen der königl. böhm. Gesellschaft der Wissenschaften* **3.** (Also appears in the Textbook of Arithmetic and Algebra.)

20. *Optisches Diastemometer, ein Instrument, wodurch man die Entfernung eines Gegenstandes durch ein blosses Anvisieren desselben augenblicklich bestimmen kann.* (The optical diastemometer, an instrument by which the distance of an object can immediately be determined by a single sighting.) Borrosch & André, Prague

21. *Über eine wesentliche Verbesserung der katoptrischen Mikroscope.* (On a significant improvement to the catoptric microscope.) Borrosch & André, Prague

22. *Über ein Mittel, periodische Bewegungen von ungemeiner Schnelligkeit noch wahrnehmbar zu machen und zu bestimmen.* (On a means of making periodic movements of extreme speed perceptible and measurable.) *Abhandlungen der königl. böhm. Gesellschaft der Wissenschaften* **3.** (Also Borrosch & André, Prague)

23. *Über eine bei jeder Rotation des Fortpflanzungsmittels mit Notwendigkeit sich einstellende eigenthümliche Ablenkung der Licht- und Schallstrahlen.* (On a characteristic deviation of light and sound waves which necessarily adjust themselves to each rotation of the propagatory medium.) *Ibid.* (Also Borrosch & André, Prague)

24. *Über die bisherigen Erklärungsversuche des Aberrations-Phänomens.* (On previous attempts to explain the phenomenon of aberration.) *Ibid.* (Also Borrosch & André, Prague)

25. *Über ein Omatogoniometer oder Gesichtswinkelmesser.* (On an omatogoniometer for measuring the visual angle.) *Ibid.*

26. *Über eine katoptrische Vorrichtung zum Abstecken der sogenannten Eisenbahnkurven und anderer krummer Linien.* (On a captoptric device to plot out the so-called railway curves and other bent lines.) *Ibid.*

1846

27. *Methode, die Geschwindigkeit, mit der die Luftmolekel beim Schalle schwingen, zu bestimmen.* (Methods to determine acoustically the speed with which the air molecules vibrate.) Borrosch & André, Prague

28. *Über ein Zerstreuungsvermögen des Fortpflanzungsmittels völlig unabhängiger rotatorischer Dispersion des Lichtes, nebst gelegentlichen Bemerkungen zur rotatorischen Brechung.* (On a rotatory dispersion of light which is completely independent of the diffusibility of the propagatory medium, and some incidental remarks on rotatory refraction.) *Ibid.*

29. *Bemerkungen zu meiner Theorie des farbigen Lichtes der Doppelsterne mit vorzüglicher Rücksicht auf die von Herrn Dr. Ballot in Utrecht dagegen erhobenen Bedenken.* (Remarks on my theory of the coloured light of the double stars, with special reference to the reservations raised against it by Dr. Ballot in Utrecht.) *Poggendorf's Annalen der Physik*, 68 **5**: 1—35

30. *Beiträge zur Fixsternenkunde.* (Contributions to knowledge of the fixed stars.) Borrosch & André, Prague. (See also nos. 31, 32 & 33 below)

1847

31. *Gedanken über die Möglichkeit, die absoluten Entfernungen und absoluten Durchmesser der Fixsterne auf rein optischem Wege zu bestimmen.* (Thoughts on the possibility of determining the absolute distances and absolute diameter of the fixed stars by purely optical means.) Borrosch & André, Prague

32. *Methode, die Geschwindigkeit, mit der die Lichtmolekel bei der Wahrnehmung der Fixsterne am Orte des Beobachters schwingen, zu bestimmen.* (Methods of determining the speed with which light molecules vibrate on the perception of the fixed stars at the position of the observer.) *Ibid.*

33. *Methode, die scheinbaren Durchmesser sämmtlicher Fixsterne im Bogenmass zu bestimmen.* (Methods to determine the apparent diameter of all fixed stars in an arc.) *Abhandlungen der königl. böhm. Gesellschaft der Wissenschaften* **4.** (Also Borresch & André, Prague)

The above three publications also appeared in "Contributions to knowledge of the fixed stars" published by Borresch & André in 1846.

34. *Über eine Vorrichtung, mittels derer sich jede noch so geringe Ablenkung eines Lichtstrahles von seiner geradlinigen Bahn wahrnehmbar machen und messen lässt, nebst Hindeutung auf solche Fälle, wo eine derartige Ablenkung vielleicht stattgefunden haben dürfte.* (On a device by means of which every minute deviation of a beam of light from its linearity can be perceived and measured, including reference to such cases where this kind of deviation has perhaps been allowed to take place.) Borresch & André, Prague

The above work was published, together with 27 and 28, under the title *Drei Abhandlungen aus dem Gebiet der Wellen-Lehre, nebst Anwendungen auf Akustik, Optik und Astronomie.* (Three works on the subject of the theory of waves, with applications in acoustics, optics and astronomy) in the *Abhandlungen der königl. böhm. Gesellschaft der Wissenschaften* (1847) 4: 497

1848

35. *Versuch einer systematischen Classification der Farben.* (An attempt at a systematic classification of the colours.) Borresch & André, Prague

36. *Über den Einfluss des Fortpflanzungsmittels auf die Erscheinungen der Aether-, Luft- und Wasserwellen, ein weiterer Beitrag zur Allgemeinen Wellenlehre.* (On the influence of the movement of the propagatory medium on the appearance of the ether, air and sound waves; a further contribution to the general theory of waves). *Abhandlungen der königl. böhm. Gesellschaft der Wissenschaften* **5.** (Also Borresch & André, Prague)

37. *Über die Anzahl der möglichen Gesichtswahrnehmungen.* (On the number of possible visual perceptions.) *Ibid.*

38. *Über eine beobachtete optische Polaritäts-Erscheinung.* (On an observed optical characteristic of polarity.) Borresch & André, Prague

39. *Versuch einer auf rein mechanischen Principien sich stützenden Erklärung der galvano-elektrischen und magnetischen Polaritätserscheinungen.* (An attempt to explain the galvano-electrical and magnetic polarity phenomena on a purely mechanical basis.) *Denkschriften d. kaiserl. Akademie d. Wissenschaften* **1.** (Also Braumüller, Vienna)
A shortened version was later (1850) published in the *Sitzungsbericht der kaiserlichen Akademie der Wissenschaften* **3**: 26

1849

40. *Über eine noch unbenützte Quelle magnetischer Declinationsbeobachtungen.* (On an as yet unused source of magnetic declination observations.) *Sitzungsbericht d. kaiserl. Akademie d. Wissenschaften* **2**: 249

41. *Über ein Mittel, die Brechung der Schallstrahlen experimentell nachzuweisen und zu bestimmen.* (On a means of experimentally proving and determining the refraction of sound waves.) *Ibid.* **2**: 322—329

42. *Über eine Reihe markscheiderischer Declinationsbeobachtungen aus der Zeit 1735—1736.* (On a series of declination observations made by surveyors of mines from 1735—1736.) *Ibid.* **3**: 1—4

43. *Über ein Mittel, die Spannkraft des Wasserdampfes der comprimierten oder erwärmten Luft durch das Gehör zu bestimmen.* (On a means of determining acoustically the pressure of water vapour in compressed or warmed air.) *Ibid.* **3**: 156—165

44. *Über eine merkwürdige in Oberösterreich aufgefundene gelatinöse Substanz.* (On a strange gelatinous substance found in Upper Austria.) *Ibid.* **3**: 239—240

1850

45. *Bemerkungen und Anträge, die magnetischen Beobachtungsdaten aus Joachimsthal, Freiburg etc. betreffend.* (Remarks and proposals concerning the magnetic observation data from Joachimsthal, Freiburg, etc.) *Ibid.* **4**: 366

46. *Einige Mittheilungen und Bemerkungen, eine Theorie des farbigen Lichtes der Doppelsterne betreffend.* (Some information and remarks concerning a theory of the coloured light of the double stars.) *Ibid.* **5**: 154

47. *Mittheilungen über ältere magnetische Declinationsbeobachtungen (Hrsg.).* (Communications on older observations of magnetic declination [Ed.].) Braumüller, Vienna

48. *Einige weitere Mittheilungen und Bemerkungen, meine Theorie des farbigen Lichtes der Doppelsterne etc. betreffend.* (Some further information and remarks concerning my theory of the coloured light of the double stars, etc.) *Poggendorf's Annalen der Physik* **81**: 270—275

1851

49. *Über die Anwendung der Syrene und des akustischen Flugrädchens zur Bestimmung des Spannungsgrades der Wasserdämpfe und der comprimirten Luft.* (On the application of the siren and the acoustic flywheel for determining the degree of pressure of water vapours and compressed air.) *Sitzungsbericht d. kaiserl. Akademie d. Wissenschaften* **6**: 206—214

50. *Über den Einfluss der Bewegung auf die Intensität der Töne etc.* (On the influence of movement on the intensity of sound, with reference to the reservations raised by Dr. Seebeck.) *Ibid.* **6**

1852

51. *Weitere Mittheilungen, meine Theorie des farbigen Lichts der Doppelsterne betreffend.* (Further information concerning my theory on the coloured light of the double stars.) *Poggendorf's Annalen der Physik* **85**: 371—378

52. *Bemerkungen zu dem Aufsatze „Über ein allgemeines Princip der Undulationslehre: Gesetz der Erhaltung der Schwingungsdauer".* (Remarks on the paper "On a general principle of the undulation theory: A law of maintenance of the wavelength". *Sitzungsbericht d. kaiserl. Akademie d. Wissenschaften* **8**: 587—593

53. *Bemerkungen über die von dem Herrn Prof. Petzval gegen die Richtigkeit meiner Theorie vorgebrachten Einwendungen.* (Remarks on the reservations raised by Prof. Petzval against the correctness of my theory.) *Ibid.* **9**: 217—255

1853

54. *Über die Möglichkeit, die Anzahl und den absoluten Abstand der Körperatome sowie das Mass ihrer wechselseitigen Anziehungsstärke zunächst bei den verschiedenen einfachen festen Körpern zu bestimmen.* (On the possibility to determine the number and the absolute distance of the atoms, as well as their reciprocal force of attraction, firstly with various simple solid bodies.) Published (1953) in the *Jahrbuch der österreichischen Akademie der Wissenschaften* 498—514

"On the Coloured Light of the Double Stars"
Facsimile Edition with English Translation

It is surprising that, until my son and I translated Doppler's famous work into the English language for my publication in 1988 (36), there appears to have been no translation into this or any other foreign language. In rectifying this omission, we decided to tamper as little as possible with the original style of the work. An early attempt to "modernise" Doppler's style by dividing up many of the lengthy sentences and deleting many of the abundance of superfluous words, in order to make it more comprehensible to today's reader, was soon abandoned. The maintenence of Doppler's style has also been attempted by avoiding words which would not been in use in the English language during the first half of the 19th century.

We did allow ourselves certain liberties, however. The first was to place Doppler's illustrative figures, which appear all together on the final page of his original publication (possibly due to the limitations of printing techniques at those times), within the part of the text to which they refer. In doing so, we followed the example of Lorentz, whose 1907 edition of selected works of Doppler (59) is certainly much easier to follow as a result of this change. A second modification is the conversion of the Austrian miles which Doppler used as a unit of distance into the English statute mile, using a factor of 4.6 and rounding off the result. It is hoped that the reader will be spared some understandable confusion by this having been done.

Several small errors in the original text have also been corrected in translation. For instance, a comparison of the German and English versions of § 4, which appear on pages 110 and 111, will show that the words *"das untere Zeichen"* (the lower representation) in the second reference to Formula (2), have been corrected to "the upper representation" in the English. Insignificant errors in numerical calculations that appear from time to time in Doppler's work have been left unchanged.

The copy of the Doppler work used in the facsimile edition is one in the possession of the University Library in Salzburg, and is dedicated by Doppler to that library — although it was the Library of the Lyceum when he presented it. In a biographical article, Andrade (2) states that the publication date of this work is usually misstated as 1842, but that it was not, in fact, published until the following year. The title page (pages 100 and 101) shows that this is not so, and that Andrade and other authors who took up his "correction" (34, 89) are themselves in error. This is due to the fact that Doppler had a small number of copies printed by Borrosch & André in Prague before its publication in the Proceedings of the Royal Bohemian Society of Sciences the following year. Doppler himself, when referring to the work, gave the reference "Prag 1842 bei Borrosch und André" (20).

Ueber das

farbige Licht der Doppelsterne

und einiger anderer

Gestirne des Himmels.

Versuch einer das Bradley'sche Aberrations-Theorem als integrirenden Theil in sich schliessenden allgemeineren Theorie.

Von

Christian Doppler,

Professor der Mathematik und praktischen Geometrie am technischen Institute und ausserordentl. Mitglied der königl. böhm. Gesellschaft der Wissenschaften.

On the

Coloured Light of the Double Stars

and Certain Other

Stars of the Heavens

An Attempt at a General Theory which Incorporates Bradley's Theorem of Aberration as an Integral Part.

by

Christian Doppler

Professor of Mathematics and Practical Geometry at the Technical Institute and Associate Member of the Royal Bohemian Society of Sciences.

From the author, to the k. k.* Lyceum Library in Salzburg as a gift.

* k. k. = Kaiserliche Königliche = Imperial & Royal

Ueber das

farbige Licht der Doppelsterne

und einiger anderer

Gestirne des Himmels.

Versuch einer das Bradley'sche Aberrations-Theorem als integrirenden Theil in sich schliessenden allgemeineren Theorie.

Von

Christian Doppler,

Professor der Mathematik und praktischen Geometrie am technischen Institute und ausserordentl. Mitglied der königl. böhm. Gesellschaft der Wissenschaften.

(Aus den Abhandlungen der k. böhm. Gesellschaft der Wissenschaften (V Folge, Bd. 2) besonders abgedruckt.)

Prag, 1842.

In Commission bei Borrosch & André.

On the

Coloured Light of the Double Stars

and Certain Other

Stars of the Heavens

An Attempt at a General Theory which Incorporates Bradley's Theorem of Aberration as an Integral Part.

by

Christian Doppler

Professor of Mathematics and Practical Geometry at the Technical Institute and Associate Member of the Royal Bohemian Society of Sciences.

(Reprinted from the Proceedings of the Royal Bohemian Society of Sciences, Vth. Ed., Vol. 2)

Prague, 1842.

In commission with Borrosch & André.

Ueber das farbige Licht der Doppelsterne und einiger anderer Gestirne des Himmels.

(Gelesen bei der königl. böhm. Gesellschaft der Wissenschaften zu Prag, in der naturwissenschaftlichen Sectionssitzung vom 25. Mai 1842.)

§. 1.

Die Undulationstheorie des Lichtes, sowie sie *Euler* und *Huygens* allererst aufstellten und mit vielem Scharfsinne gegen die erklärtesten Gegner derselben vertheidigten, ist im Verlaufe ihrer weitern Ausbildung bekanntlich auf Schwierigkeiten gestossen, welche spätere ausgezeichnete Gelehrte, wie *Young*, *Fresnel*, *Cauchy* u. A. dahin vermochten, von der ursprünglichen, wie es scheint nur allein naturgemässen und einfachen Voraussetzung sphärischer oder longitudinaler Aetherschwingungen abzugehen und sich zur Annahme blosser derartiger transversaler Schwingungen zu verstehen. Die glänzenden Erfolge dieser neuen Voraussetzung haben seitdem auch mehrere derjenigen Physiker, wenn auch nicht eben überzeugt doch vorläufig einigermassen beruhigt, welche sich von allem Anfange her nur höchst ungern und mit sichtlichem Widerstreben dieser neuen Ansicht über die Natur des Lichtes hingaben. Und so ist es denn gekommen, dass während diese Ansicht den feinsten analytischen Untersuchungen fortwährend zum Grunde gelegt wird, und zu mehr oder minder glücklichen Resultaten führet, man die Untersuchung und jegliche Discussion über die Zulässigkeit und innere Wahrscheinlichkeit dieser neuen Hypothese vor der Hand so gut wie fallen liess. Auf eine vollständige und erschöpfende Erklärung sämmtlicher bisher bekannter Lichterscheinungen nach diesem Prinzipe, scheint es, wolle man es ankommen lassen, diese wolle man abwarten, und sodann erst versuchen, ob man sich mit wahrhafter Ueberzeugung dieser neuen Voraussetzung zuzuwenden vermögen wird.

Indessen giebt es bekanntlich sehr viele, die, wiewohl sie den Werth analytischer Ergebnisse in vollem Masse zu würdigen wissen, gleichwohl einen derartigen durchaus glücklichen Erfolg noch sehr bezweifeln und geradezu auf die Schwierigkeiten aufmerksam machen,

On the Coloured Light of the Double Stars and Certain Other Stars of the Heavens.

(Read at the Royal Bohemian Society for Sciences in Prague, in the Meeting of the Section of Natural Sciences of 25th. May 1842)

§ 1

The undulatory theory of light, first put forward by *Euler* and *Huygens* and astutely defended against its most proclaimed opponents, has obviously run into difficulties in the course of its further development, inducing later distinguished scholars such as *Young, Fresnel, Cauchy* and others, to abandon the original – and apparently only natural and simple – idea of spherical or longitudinal ether waves, in favour of transverse waves of that nature. The brilliant success of this new premise has since, if not completely convinced, certainly somewhat temporarily reassured those physicists who from the beginning accepted this new view of the nature of light only reluctantly and with visible resistance. And now that this view has since been continuously subjected to the finest analytical examination with more or less favourable results, any discussion about the feasibility or high probability of this new hypothesis has been as good as dropped. It appears that one must await a complete and exhaustive explanation of all known manifestations of light according to this principle, and only then can one judge if these new postulates can be embraced with true conviction.

It is also well known that there are very many who, although they fully respect the value of analytical conclusions, still strongly doubt such a completely favourable outcome and point out the

1*

denen im steigenden Masse diese neuere Theorie entgegen gehet*). — *Laplace* und *Poisson*, welchem Letzteren die Lichttheorie so viel verdanket, waren bekanntlich bis zum letzten Augenblicke ganz entschieden gegen diese neue Modification der Undulationstheorie, und haben diese ihre Ueberzeugung, wo sich nur immer die Gelegenheit hierzu darbot, mit Offenheit und ohne allen Rückhalt ausgesprochen. Auch *Herschel* d. j. hält diese Ansicht über die Natur des Lichtes (man sehe dessen Werk über das Licht, S. 540) durchaus noch nicht für die richtige und wahre, und er scheint sie nur einstweilen, ihrer Erfolge wegen, mehr dulden als vertheidigen und pflegen zu wollen. Dieser Meinung scheinen auch *Brandes* und viele andere höchst achtbare Physiker der Jetztzeit zu seyn, und es ist überhaupt sehr die Frage, ob nicht selbst die eigentlichen Vertheidiger der transversalen Schwingungen, wenn sie von den glücklichen Resultaten ihres Calcüls absehen, eingestehen müssen, dass man zu dieser ihrer Voraussetzung einen etwas starken Glauben mitzubringen habe. Es ist aber hier nicht an der Zeit, zu erörtern, wie hoch überhaupt der Werth einiger oder auch vieler mit der Erfahrung gut stimmender Rechnungsresultate gegenüber einer Voraussetzung anzuschlagen ist, die, wie es wenigstens dem Verfasser dieser Zeilen scheint, den Charakter einer grossen innern Unwahrscheinlichkeit an sich trägt. Wie immer aber auch in der Zukunft der Streit hierüber ausgetragen werden mag, so kann unter so bewandten Umständen wohl niemand sich vorzugsweise aufgefordert fühlen, irgend eine optische Naturerscheinung eben gerade nach dem Prinzipe der Lateral-Schwingungen erklären zu wollen.

§. 2.

Nach der ursprünglichen Vibrationshypothese ist bekanntlich die Farbempfindung eine unmittelbare Folge der in gewissen Zeitintervallen regelmässig aufeinanderfolgenden Pulsationen oder Wellenschläge des Aethers. Die Intensität des farbigen Lichtes dagegen hängt lediglich von der Grösse der Excursionen jedes einzelnen Aethertheilchens oder beziehungsweise derjenigen ab, welche unmittelbar die Retina des Auges berühren. Alles, was demnach das Intervall der Zeit, die zwischen den einzelnen Stössen des Aethers verfliesst, ändert, zieht nothwendig eine Aenderung der Farbe nach sich, und jeder Umstand, der bewirket, dass die einzelnen Wellenschläge mit verminderter oder vermehrter Energie erfolgen, ändert den Inten-

*) Das Aberrations-Phänomen als solches darf wohl heut zu Tage, wo es bis auf die feinsten Details durchgeprüft erscheint, für fast eben so constatirt angesehen werden, wie irgend eine andere Erscheinung in der Lehre vom Lichte. Unter Voraussetzung longitudinaler Aetherschwingungen bietet die Erklärung desselben nicht die geringste Schwierigkeit dar, ja folgt mit Nothwendigkeit aus der Zusammensetzung der Aetherwellen mit der eigenen fortschreitenden Bewegung der Erde. Nicht aber lässt sich ein Gleiches bei Annahme transversaler Schwingungen behaupten. *Fresnel*, der Mitbegründer der neueren Undulationslehre, hat dieses bekanntlich selbst anerkannt. Aber nicht nur nicht zu erklären vermag man dieses Phänomen nach dieser Voraussetzung; sondern es scheint sogar mit der neuern Undulationslehre in einem offenbaren und directen Widerspruche zu stehen. Sollte hierin für die eigentlichen Vertreter dieser Lehre nicht eine sehr bestimmte Aufforderung liegen, die Zulänglichkeit ihres Prinzipes vor Allem an der Erklärung dieser Erscheinung zu erproben? — Bis dahin aber, wo dieses geschehen seyn wird, dürfte wohl auch unserm gegenwärtigen Erklärungsversuche die gleiche billige Beachtung und Prüfung kaum versagt werden können. —

difficulties which confront this newer theory to an increasing degree*). – *Laplace* and *Poisson,* to whom the theory of light owes so much, were decidedly opposed to the very last against this new modification of the undulatory theory and – as is well known – voiced their convictions frankly and without reserve whenever the opportunity presented itself. Also *Herschel* the younger does not yet hold this view of the nature of light (see his work on light, p. 540) by any means to be the correct and true one, and he appears for the time being to tolerate it due to its success rather than to defend and to subscribe to it. This opinion also seems to be held by *Brandes* and many other highly respected physicists of our time, and the question is allowed as to whether even the very defenders of transverse waves, putting aside the fortunate results of their calculations, must admit that the acceptance of their ideas requires a great deal of faith. This is not the time to consider how high the values of a few, or even of many, with good mathematical results can be set against a supposition which appears, at least to the author of these lines, to bear the characteristics of a great inner uncertainty. However this dispute might be resolved in the future, under such circumstances no one can feel particularly qualified to explain any optical phenomenon according to the principle of lateral waves.

§ 2

According to the original hypothesis of vibration, it is known that perception of colour is a direct result of pulsations or waves of the ether which occur at certain regular intervals. The intensity of the coloured light, on the other hand, depends solely on the size of the excursion of each single ether particle, or rather those that directly touch the retina of the eye. Everything that changes the time interval between the single impacts of the ether, necessarily brings a change of colour with it and every circumstance that causes the single wave impacts to occur with reduced or increased energy,

*) The aberration phenomenon as such may well be viewed today, having been tested down to the finest detail, as established as any other in the study of light. The acceptance of longitudinal ether waves does not pose the slightest problem, indeed is a necessary result of the composition of the ether waves with the increasing movement of the Earth. The same, however, cannot be said about the acceptance of transverse waves. *Fresnel,* the co-founder of the newer school of undulation, has himself recognised this. But it is not only its inability to explain this phenomenon under these circumstances; rather that it even appears to stand in an obvious and direct opposition to the new school of undulation. Should this not present a challenge for the true advocates of this doctrine to test the adequacy of their principle above all on the explanation of this appearance? – Until this happens, our own present explanatory attempts cannot be denied equal and fair consideration and examination. –

sitätsgrad des farbigen und weissen Lichtes. Letzteres hängt wieder damit zusammen, dass in diesem Falle die Grösse der Excursionen, welche jedes Aetherteilchen macht, sich ändert. Was hier von den Lichtwellen gesagt und behauptet wurde, gilt natürlich auch vollkommen strenge von den Schallwellen, und man hat daher auch von jeher bis zu dem oben bezeichneten Zeitpunkte die verschiedenen Lichtphänomene aus jenen des Schalles auf dem Wege der Analogie mit vielem Glücke zu erklären gesucht. — Es dünkt mich aber sehr bemerkenswerth, dass man sowohl in der Licht- und Schall-Lehre, wie auch in der allgemeinen Wellenlehre meines Wissens wenigstens auf einen möglicher Weise sehr wohl vorkommenden Umstand bisher so gut wie keine Rücksicht genommen hat! Es scheint nämlich, man habe völlig unbeachtet gelassen, dass, wenn man von den Licht- und Schallwellen als Ursachen der Licht- und Schallempfindungen und nicht bloss als von objectiven Vorgängen spricht, man nicht sowohl darnach fragen müsse, in welchen Zeiträumen und mit welchen Intensitätsgraden die Wellenerzeugung an und für sich vor sich gehe, — als vielmehr darnach, in welchen Zeitintervallen und mit welcher Stärke diese Aether- oder Luftschwingungen vom Auge oder vom Ohre irgend eines Beobachters aufgenommen und empfunden werden. Von diesen rein subjectiven Bestimmungen, nicht aber von dem objectiven Sachverhalte hängt die Farbe und Intensität einer Lichtempfindung oder die Tonhöhe und Stärke irgend eines Schalles ab. Ereignet es sich daher irgend wie, dass eine numerische Verschiedenheit zwischen dem objectiven Vorgange und dem subjectiven Ergebnisse sich hierbei herausstellt: so hat man sich ganz unzweifelhaft an die subjectiven Bestimmungen zu halten. Im ersten Augenblicke mag es nun freilich scheinen, als sey das Gesagte mehr für eine bloss gelehrte Distinction, denn für eine von wichtigen praktischen Folgen begleitete Bemerkung zu halten. Doch hierüber möge der geehrte Leser, sobald er die nachfolgenden Zeilen einiger Erwägung gewürdiget, selbst entscheiden. — So lange man nämlich voraussetzet, dass sowohl der Beobachter als auch die Quelle der Wellen unverändert ihren anfänglichen Ort beibehalten, unterliegt es freilich keinem weitern Zweifel, dass die subjectiven Bestimmungen mit den objectiven numerisch vollkommen zusammenfallen werden. Wie aber, wenn entweder der Beobachter oder die Quelle oder gar beide zugleich ihren Ort veränderten, sich von einander entfernten oder sich einander näherten, und dieses zwar mit einer Geschwindigkeit, die mit jener, nach der die Wellen fortschreiten, in einigen Vergleich käme? Dürfte auch in diesem Falle auf eine solche Uebereinstimmung beider zu rechnen seyn? Ich glaube kaum, dass der Leser sich geneigt fühlen dürfte, diese Frage ohne eine vorgängige Untersuchung geradezu zu bejahen! — In der That scheint nichts begreiflicher, als dass der Weg und die Zwischenzeit zweier aufeinanderfolgender Wellenschläge für einen Beobachter sich verkürzen muss, wenn der Beobachter der ankommenden Welle entgegeneilt, und verlängern, wenn er ihr enteilt, und dass auch gleichzeitig im ersteren Falle die Intensität des Wellenschlags grösser werden, im zweiten dagegen nothwendig sich vermindern muss. Bei einer Bewegung der Wellenquelle selbst findet natürlich eine ähnliche Veränderung in demselben Sinne statt. Hat doch auch der gemeinen Erfahrung zufolge ein auch nur etwas tiefgehendes Schiff, welches den andringenden Wellen gerade entgegensteuert, in derselben Zeit eine grössere Anzahl und viel heftigere

changes the degree of intensity of the coloured and white light. The latter is further related to the changes in the size of the excursion made by each ether particle. What is said and claimed here for light waves naturally also applies to sound waves, and one has therefore tried with considerable success – from time immemorial until the juncture referred to above – to explain the various phenomena of light by means of analogies with sound. But it seems remarkable to me that in the science of both light and sound, as well as in the general theory of waves, one has – at least as far as I know – failed to take into consideration one commonly occuring circumstance! It seems that the fact has been ignored that in speaking of light and sound waves as being the causes of light and sound perception and not merely as objective processes, one should not so much ask in what space of time and with what level of intensity the creation of waves actually takes place but rather at which time intervals and with what strength these ether or air waves are picked up and perceived by the eye or ear of the observer. It is from these purely subjective conditions, and not from the objective facts, that the colour and intensity of light-perception or the pitch and volume of any sound are dependent. If by any chance a numerical difference should occur between the objective process and the subjective results, then one must without any doubt adhere to the subjective evaluation. At the first glance it may well appear as though what has been said above is of merely academic distinction rather than observations that are accompanied by practical consequences. On this point the honoured reader, as soon as he has given the following lines his worthy consideration, shall decide for himself. – So long as it is assumed that the observer, as well as the source of the waves, remain in their original position without moving, there can be no doubt that the subjective evaluation will numerically coincide completely with the objective. What, however, if either the observer or the source – or even both together – change their position, move away from or nearer to each other, and this with a speed comparable to that with which the waves are propagated? Could also in this case such a conformity be reckoned with? I hardly believe that the reader could feel inclined to give an affirmative answer to this question without previous investigation! – In fact, nothing seems easier to comprehend than that the distance and time interval between two successive waves must become shorter for an observer who is hurrying towards the oncoming waves and longer if he is moving away, and similarly, in the first case the intensity of the wave is stronger and in the second it must necessarily decrease. With a movement of the source of the waves itself, a similar change naturally takes place in the same sense. We know from general experience that a ship with a moderately deep draught which is steering towards the oncoming waves has to

Wellenschläge zu erleiden, wie eines, das ruhet oder gar sich in der Richtung der Wellen mit ihnen fortbewegt. Was aber von den Wasserwellen gilt, warum dürfte dieses nicht mit den nöthigen Modificationen auch von den Luft- und Aetherwellen angenommen werden? Es scheint, als ob sich dagegen etwas Erhebliches kaum vorbringen lassen dürfte! — Unter diesen Umständen mag es zweckdienlich scheinen, die nöthigen darauf bezüglichen, ganz einfachen Formeln aufzustellen, und indem wir dieselben versuchsweise auf die Schallwellen anwenden, glauben wir zugleich auch der Akustik einen kleinen Dienst zu erweisen.

§. 3.

Wenn Beobachter und Wellenquelle sich einander nähern oder von einander entfernen, so kann die Richtung ihrer Bewegung, falls sie eine geradlinige ist, in ihre Verbindungslinie fallen, oder ihre Richtungen schliessen einen Winkel ein. Alles, was dabei eine Aenderung erfahren kann, ist die Dauer zwischen den aufeinander folgenden Wellenschlägen, ihre Intensität und die Richtung, in der sie dem Beobachter anzukommen scheinen. Der letztere Punkt kömmt bei unserer gegenwärtigen Untersuchung nicht in Betracht, und ist überdiess schon durch *Bradley's* scharfsinniges Aberrations-Theorem als erledigt anzusehen. Es bleibt uns demnach nur der erstere Fall einer directen Annäherung oder Entfernung für die Betrachtung übrig, wo die Frage über die Richtung nicht zur Sprache kömmt. Diesen vorliegenden Fall dagegen müssen wir unter einer doppelten Voraussetzung betrachten; das einemal nämlich, wo der Beobachter in Bewegung und die Quelle in Ruhe, das anderemal, wo gerade das Gegentheil davon angenommen wird.

Fall 1. Es heisse die Geschwindigkeit, mit welcher die Wellen fortgepflanzt werden, a, und O und A (Fig. 1 und 2) bedeute Anfang und Ende einer Welle, Q dagegen die entfernte Quelle derselben; ferner n die Anzahl Sekunden, die eine Welle nöthig hat, um von A nach O zu kommen, d. h. um eine Wellenlänge zu durchlaufen, und x'' die Zeit, die sie braucht, um den gegen oder von A sich bewegenden Beobachter O zu erreichen. Man hat daher für den Fall der Annäherung sowohl wie der Entfernung des Beobachters von oder an die Quelle, wegen $a x'' \pm \alpha x = a n''$; 1, $x'' = \frac{a n}{a \pm \alpha}$; oder auch $\alpha = \pm\left(1 - \frac{n''}{x''}\right) a$

Fall 2. Wenn dagegen der Beobachter unbeweglich ist, die Quelle sich dagegen mit der Geschwindigkeit α zu oder von dem Beobachter bewegt: so hat man vor Allem den Einfluss dieser Bewegung auf die der Quelle nächste Welle zu berücksichtigen, da die einzelnen entstandenen Wellen, wie Fig. 3 und 4 veranschaulicht, in völlig unveränderter Weise bis zum entfernten Beobachter in O fortgepflanzt werden. Während daher die erste Welle von Q nach A gelangt, wobei sie einen Weg gleich $a n$ durchläuft, ist die Quelle Q selbst nach Q' gekommen, wobei sie einen Weg gleich αn macht, und die zweite Welle braucht nur noch eben so viele Zeit, als zum Durchlaufen der entsprechenden Wellenlänge $Q'A$ nöthig ist. Man hat daher für beide Fälle, wegen $a n'' \mp \alpha n'' = a x''$, 2, $x = \left(\frac{a \mp \alpha}{a}\right) n$; oder auch

$$\alpha = \pm\left(\frac{x}{n} - 1\right) a.$$

receive, in the same amount of time, more waves with a greater impact compared with a ship that is not moving or is even travelling along on the direction of the waves. If this should be valid for waves of water, then why should it not also be applied with necessary modifications to air and ether waves? It hardly seems that anything of consequence could be raised against this! – Under the circumstances it might seem expendient to set out the very simple formulae that are necessary for this and, by experimentally applying them to sound waves, we think that we could at the same time be of some small service to acoustics.

§ 3

When observer and wave-source move nearer to or away from each other, the direction of their movement, so long as it forms a straight line, is on the line connecting them, or their directions form an angle. All that can produce a change is the time between the consecutive waves, their intensity and the direction from which they appear to approach the observer. The latter point is not relevant to our present investigation and is, moreover, considered as settled by *Bradley's* perspicacious theorum of aberration. Therefore there remains only the first case of a direct drawing nearer or moving apart for us to consider, in which the question of direction does not require discussion. The case in question on the other hand, we must view under a double set of conditions: the first in which the observer is in motion and the source is stationary, and the other in which exactly the opposite applies.
Case 1. In which the speed with which the waves are propagated, a, and O and A (Figs. 1 & 2) indicate the beginning and end of the wave, Q on the other hand is the distant source of these; further n represents the number of seconds that a wave takes to come from A to O, i.e., to travel through a wavelength, and x'' for the time that it needs to reach the observer O who is travelling to or from A. In the case of the observer moving either towards or away from the source, thus

$$ax'' \pm \alpha x'' = an; \quad (1)$$

$$x'' = \frac{an}{a \pm \alpha}; \quad \text{or also} \quad \alpha = \pm\left(1 - \frac{n''}{x''}\right) a$$

Case 2. If, on the other hand, the observer is stationary and the source is travelling towards or away from him with the speed α, one must above all take into account the influence of this movement on the wave closest to the source, because the individual waves, as Figs. 3 & 4 illustrate, are propagated in a completely unchanged way towards the distant observer O. Hence, while the first wave travels from Q to A, covering the distance equivalent to an, the source Q itself has arrived at Q', covering a distance equivalent to αn, and the second wave takes only as much time as is necessary to cover the corresponding wavelength $Q'A$. One has for both cases, thus

$$an'' \mp \alpha n'' = ax'', \quad (2) \quad x = \left(\frac{Q \mp \alpha}{a}\right) n; \quad \text{or also}$$

$$\alpha = \pm\left(\frac{x}{n} - 1\right) a.$$

Fig. 1

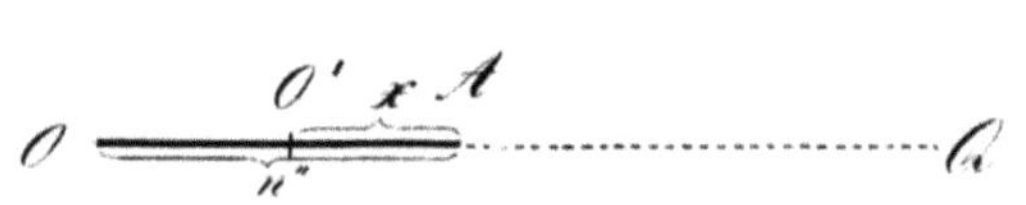

Fig. 2

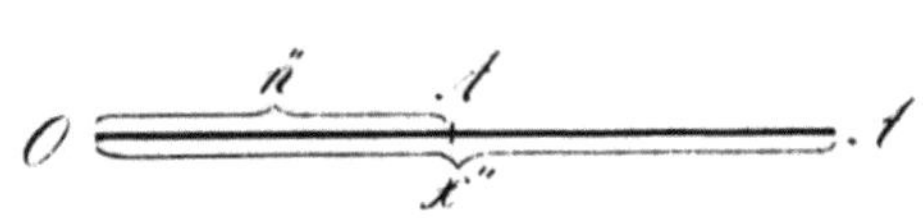

Aus der Verschiedenheit der beiden Formeln (1) und (2) ersieht man, dass es keineswegs selbst unter solchen gleichen Umständen einerlei ist, ob der Beobachter oder die Wellenquelle sich bewegt. — Rücksichtlich der Intensitätsänderung müssen wir uns, da bis jetzt die Vibrationsgeschwindigkeit der einzelnen Theilchen sich noch nicht ermitteln liess, mit der schon im Frühern ausgesprochenen allgemeinen Bemerkung begnügen. —

§. 4.

Entfernt sich der Beobachter von dem schallenden oder leuchtenden Objecte mit einer dem a selbst gleichen Geschwindigkeit, so findet man, da in Formel (1) das untere Zeichen zu gelten hat, $x = \infty$, d h. die einzelnen Schallwellen erreichen niemals das Ohr des Beobachters, und die Tonerzeugung, wiewohl an und für sich vorhanden, ist für die Wahrnehmung des Beobachters so gut wie gar nicht da. Entfernt sich aber dagegen die Tonquelle selbst mit derselben Geschwindigkeit vom Beobchter, so findet man (da in Formel (2) das untere Zeichen zu gelten hat) $x = 2n$; d. h. der Beobachter vernimmt die nächst tiefere Octav desjenigen Tones, welchen an und für sich der schallende Körper hervorbringt. — Nimmt man endlich an, dass sich die Quelle dem Beobachter mit einer Geschwindigkeit annähert, die jener der fortschreitenden Wellen selbst gleich kömmt: so hat man, da in Formel (2) das untere Zeichen zu gelten hat, wegen $a = \alpha$, $x = \frac{O \,.\, n}{a} = O$, d. h. die einzelnen Wellenschläge treffen alle im nämlichen Augenblicke beim Beobachter ein, oder was dasselbe ist, in unendlich kurzen Zeitintervallen, welcher Umstand einen unendlich hohen Ton, der gar nicht mehr vernehmbar wird, begründen würde. — Um auf einige ganz spezielle numerische Beispiele überzugehen, werde vorausgesetzt, die Geschwindigkeit des Schalles bei 10° Reaumur, d. i. a, sey 1024 par. Fuss, und man frage z. B. um die Geschwindigkeit α, mit der sich ein Beobachter gegen die Schallquelle bewegen muss, damit er das sogenannte grosse C als D vernehme, so erhält man wegen $n = \frac{1}{64}$, $x = \frac{1}{72}$, und $a = 1024$ nach Formel (1); $\alpha = 128'$ als Geschwindigkeit in der Sekunde. Umgekehrt zeigt die nämliche Formel, dass sich der Beobachter mit einer Geschwindigkeit von 114 Fuss in der Sekunde von der Schallquelle entfernen müsste, damit das D als grosses C vernommen würde. Noch viel günstiger für die Wahrnehmung irgend einer Tonänderung sind andere sich näher liegende Töne, da sie bei absoluter gleicher Fortpflanzungsgeschwindigkeit des Schalles dennoch einander näher liegende Schwingungszahlen darbieten. So z.. B bedarf es, wegen $n = \frac{1}{120}$ und $x = \frac{1}{128}$ und $a = 1024$ nur einer Geschwindigkeit $\alpha = 68'$ von Seite eines Beobachters, um den Ton H als c zu vernehmen. Ein geübtes Ohr unterscheidet aber bekanntlich Tonunterschiede bis auf einen Viertelton, und es bedürfte daher gar nur nach Formel (1) einer Geschwindigkeit α von kaum 17′ in der Sekunde, um bei dem Tone H eine Erhöhung oder auch Erniedrigung von einem Viertelton zu bewirken. Berücksichtigt man nun, dass die Annäherung oder das Entfernen ein wechselseitiges seyn kann, so ist der Fall gar nicht undenkbar, wo bei einer beiderseitigen

Fig. 3

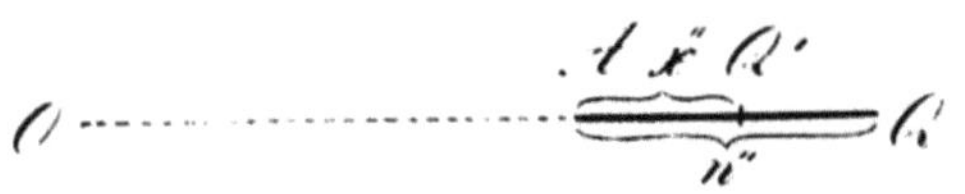

Fig. 4

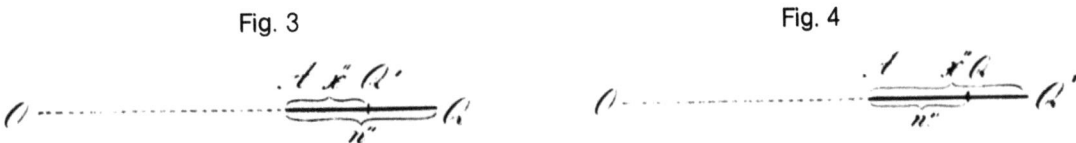

From the difference between the two Formulae (1) and (2) one sees that, even under such similar conditions, it is by no means the same if the observer or if the source is moving. – With regard to the change in intensity, since the vibration speed of the individual particles has not yet been determined we must be content with the general comments voiced earlier. –

§ 4

If the observer moves away with a constant speed, equal to *a*, from the object which is emitting sound or light then, since the lower representation of Formula (1) is valid, that $x = \infty$, i.e., individual sound waves never reach the ear of the observer and the source of the sound, although present, is for the perception of the observer as good as not there at all. If, however, the source of sound itself is moving away from the observer at the same speed it will be found (since in Formula (2) the lower representation is valid) $x = 2n$, i.e., the observer perceives the next lower octave of that note which is actually produced by the source. If it is lastly presumed that the source is moving towards the observer with a speed that is equal to the speed of the waves themselves, since in Formula (2) the upper representation is valid, thus, $\alpha = a$, $x = \frac{O \cdot n}{a} = O$ i.e., the individual waves arrive at the observer at the same time or at infinitely short time intervals, both of which would result in an infinitely high note which would be impossible to hear. – Turning to a number of very specific numerical examples, it is assumed that the speed of sound at 10 Reaumur, viz. *a*, is 1 024 par. feet, and one may ask, for example, about the speed at which the observer would have to travel towards the sound source in order to perceive the so-called C as D, so when $n = \frac{1}{64}$, $x = \frac{1}{72}$; and $a = 1\,024$, according to Formula (1); one arrives at $\alpha = 128'$ as speed in the second. Conversely, this formula shows that the observer would have to move away from the source of sound at a speed of 114 feet in the second in order to perceive D as C. Much more favourable for a perception of a change in tone are other notes which are closer to each other, since they demonstrate a greater number of closely adjacent waves at an identical velocity of propagation of the sound. For example, where $n = \frac{1}{120}$ and $x = \frac{1}{128}$ and $a = 1024$, a speed of only $\alpha = 68'$ is needed from the part of an observer in order to perceive the note B as c. A trained ear can supposedly distinguish sounds down to a quartertone, and it therefore requires according to Formula (1) a speed α of hardly 17' in the second to produce a rise or fall of a quartertone in the note B. If one now considers that the moving together or apart can be done by both sides, then

Geschwindigkeit von nur wenigen, höchstens 8 Fuss in der Sekunde, für einen aufmerksamen Beobachter bereits kleine Tonveränderungen wahrnehmbar werden können. — Doch, ich will nun meinem vorgesteckten Ziele näher rücken, indem ich sofort die oben aufgestellten Formeln auf die Erscheinungen des Lichtes anwende.

§. 5.

Setzt man die Geschwindigkeit des Lichtes $a = 42000$ Meilen in der Sekunde, und frägt man, mit welcher Geschwindigkeit ein im weissen oder violetten Lichte leuchtendes Object sich von einem Beobachter entfernen müsse, damit es für ihn völlig unsichtbar werde, so hat man für $\frac{1}{n} = 727$ Billionen und für $\frac{1}{x} = 458$ Billionen zu setzen, und man findet für α aus Formel (2) die Geschwindigkeit von 19000 Meilen in der Sekunde. Bei einer solchen Geschwindigkeit des leuchtenden Gegenstandes würden daher, falls er sich von uns entfernte, die äussersten violetten und um so mehr alle übrigen farbigen Strahlen, folglich auch das aus ihnen zusammengesetzte weisse Licht, wäre es selbst noch so intensiv, für jede Beobachtung völlig verlöschen. Rücksichtlich der übrigen Farben reicht übrigens schon eine bedeutend geringere Geschwindigkeit zum völligen Verlöschen desselben hin. Die Formel (2) gibt nämlich für gelbes Licht die Geschwindigkeit von 5007 Meilen in der Sekunde, für rothes gar nur 1700 Meilen. Bei den hier namhaft gemachten Geschwindigkeiten würde, da immer je eine oder gar zwei der prismatischen Hauptfarben, sey es nun aus dem untern (beim Entfernen) oder aus dem obern (beim Annähern) des Spectrums ganz austritt, das zurückbleibende farbige Licht stets ein vollkommen homogenes seyn, ein Umstand, der hier sehr wohl zu beachten ist. —

Ganz anders dagegen stellt sich der Calcül, sobald wir von der Voraussetzung ausgehen, dass das beobachtete farbige Licht, weit entfernt, ein homogenes zu seyn, vielmehr ein mit vielem Weiss gemischtes ist, welcher Fall eben bei den vorliegenden Betrachtungen eintritt. *Herschel* d. j. spricht es selbst aus, dass alles mit besonders lebhaftem Glanze und grossem sogenannten Feuer leuchtende farbige Licht stets ein mit ziemlich vielen weissen Strahlen gemischtes sey, und an einem andern Orte seines vortrefflichen Werkes über das Licht nimmt er an, dass das menschliche Auge noch Farbunterschiede gewahr zu werden vermag, welche durch ein Entziehen von nur dem hunderten Theile derjenigen rothen, gelben oder blauen Strahlen hervorgehen, die mit den übrigen zu weissem Lichte sich zusammengesetzt finden. Ein weiterer sehr bemerkenswerther Umstand ist folgender. Da nämlich die Intensität oder Menge der verschiedenfarbigen Lichtstrahlen mit ihren Schwingungszahlen nicht in gleichem Verhältnisse steht, indem die im weissen Lichte enthaltenen blauen die rothen um vielleicht dreimal, die gelben sie gar um mehr als zehnmal übertreffen, und da es ferner gerade die gelben Strahlen sind, die einerseits (bei einer Annäherung) in blaue, andererseits dagegen (bei einem Entfernen) in rothe übergehen: so ist klar, dass selbst bei einer Verminderung von nur einem Hundertel der äussersten rothen oder blauen Strahlen eine wenigstens dreimal, im andern Fall sogar zehnmal grössere Anzahl von farbigen Strahlen wirksam auf-

the case is not so unthinkable whereby a speed of only a few – not more than 8 – feet in the second from each side could produce a small change in pitch which could be already detected by an alert observer. – However, I will now move closer to the goal I have set myself and will immediately apply the above calculations to the phenomena of light.

§ 5

If one sets the speed of light $a = 193\,000$ miles in the second and then asks at what speed an object emitting white or violet light must travel away from the observer so that it becomes completely invisible for him, so one has $\frac{1}{n} = 727$ billion and for $\frac{1}{x} = 458$ billion and one finds for α from Formula (2) the speed of 84 000 miles in the second. At such a speed of the light-emitting object, if it were moving away from us, the extreme violet and more so all other coloured radiations, and consequently the white light that these together produce, will become completely extinguished for every observer, no matter how bright they are. Concerning the other colours, a significantly lesser speed is adequate to extinguish these fully. Formula (2) gives a speed of 23 032 miles in the second for yellow light and only 7 820 miles for red. At the speeds named here, since one or even two of the prismatic primary colours totally disappear from the spectrum, be it from the lower end (retreating) or from the upper end (approaching) the remaining coloured light would be continuously homogeneous, a fact that is worthy of attention here. –

The calculation becomes different if we assume that the observed coloured light, far from being homogeneous, is actually mixed with much white, as is the case in the present observation. *Herschel* the younger himself says that all particularly lively brightness and the so-called fire-emitting coloured light, far from being homogeneous, is actually mixed with a good deal of white rays. At another part in his excellent work on light he postulates that the human eye is capable of registering differences in colour which result from the reduction of only a hundredth part of the those red, yellow or blue rays which, combined with the others, form white light. A further fact worthy of mention is the following. Since the intensity and quantity of the differently coloured light rays does not stand in direct relation to the number of waves, the blue rays which are contained in white light exceed the red ones by perhaps three, the yellow ones even by more than ten, and because it is just the yellow rays which on the one hand (approaching) turn to blue and on the other (retreating) to red, it is clear that with a reduction of only one hundredth of the outermost blue or red rays, there will be at least a tripling, and in

treten und eine schon sehr merkliche Färbung zu bewirken vermögen werden. Aus eben diesem Umstande folgt, dass die rothe und orange Färbung unter übrigens gleichen Umständen intensiver und dem homogenen gleichnamigen Lichte näher kommen werde, wie die blaue und grüne, und ebenso dass zur grünen, orangen oder violetten Färbung keineswegs nothwendig alle blauen, rothen oder gelben Strahlen, sondern nur einige wenige derselben auszutreten haben, da die übrigen wieder zu weissem Lichte sich vereinigen.

Diess vorausgesetzt findet man, wenn $x = \frac{1}{458}$ und $n = \frac{1}{458{\cdot}37}$ gesetzt wird, wobei also die rothen Strahlen von der Schwingungszahl 458·37 Billionen auf 458 Billionen herabgebracht werden, also der hundertste Theil der rothen Strahlen austreten, $\alpha = 33$ Meilen für die Sekunde, d. h. wenn ein im weissen Lichte leuchtender Stern sich einem Beobachter mit einer Geschwindigkeit von 33 Meilen in der Sekunde annähert oder sich von ihm entfernt, so erscheint er demselben im ersteren Falle schon merklich grün, im andern dagegen orange gefärbt. Dieser Zahlwerth dürfte auch so ziemlich als die untere Grenze gelten. Bei der Voraussetzung, dass ein ganzes Zehntel der rothen oder blauen Strahlen austreten, wodurch zu Folge der oben ausgesprochenen Umstände eine sehr starke Färbung eintreten muss, erhält man wegen $x = \frac{1}{458}$, und $n = \frac{1}{460}$, für $\alpha = 187$ Meilen in der Sekunde. — Dem Gesagten zufolge gehen daher bei einem Entfernen die im weissen Lichte enthaltenen Strahlen in solche von längerer Schwingungsdauer, also die violetten in blaue, die blauen durch grün in gelbe, die gelben durch orange in rothe über, und die rothen treten endlich bei zunehmender Geschwindigkeit ganz und gar aus, d. h. werden insensibel. Im umgekehrten Falle dagegen, wo zuerst die blauen Strahlen ausscheiden, erscheint das weisse Licht anfänglich grün, hierauf blau und endlich violett. —

§. 6.

Das bisher über den Einfluss der Bewegung auf die Lichterscheinungen Vorgebrachte lässt sich übersichtlich in nachfolgende Punkte zusammenfassen:

1. Wenn ein leuchtendes Object, gleichviel ob selbstleuchtend oder bloss beleuchtet, sich mit einer gegen die Geschwindigkeit des Lichtes in Betracht kommenden Schnelligkeit in directer Richtung dem Auge eines Beobachters nähert oder sich von ihm entfernt: so hat diese Bewegung nothwendig eine Aenderung in der Farbe und Intensität des Lichtes zur Folge und zwar:

   α. Bei einer Annäherung nimmt die Intensität jedenfalls zu, die Färbung dagegen geht bei steigender Geschwindigkeit von Weiss in Grün, von da in Blau und endlich in Violett über.

   β. Bei einem Entfernen vermindert sich dessen Intensität in jedem Falle und das weisse Licht geht allmählig in Gelb, Orange und endlich in Rroth über. Hat indessen das Licht bereits schon eine gewisse Färbung, z. B. eine gelbe, so beginnt die Veränderung von dieser an und steigt auf- und abwärts nach den in α und β ausgesprochenen Bedingungen.

the other case a tenfold amount of coloured rays that will appear and already result in a noticable coloration. From these facts it follows that the red and the orange colorations, under otherwise similar conditions, become more intensive and approach closer to the homogeneous light of the same name, just like the blue and the green, and also the blue, red or yellow rays which are by no means all necessary for green, orange or violet coloration since only a few of these have to be extinguished, the remainder recombining to form white light.

Bearing this in mind, it will be found, when $x = \frac{1}{458}$ and $n = \frac{1}{458 \cdot 37}$ so that the vibration rate of the red rays is reduced from 458.37 billions to 458 billions and thus a hundredth of the rays are extinguished, $a = 152$ miles in the second, i.e., a star radiating white light which is approaching or retreating from the observer at a speed of 152 miles in the second appears to him to be noticably green in the first case and orange-coloured in the second. This numerical value can be regarded as approximately the lower limit. Supposing that a whole tenth of the red or blue rays are extinguished which, based on the facts discussed above, must result in a very strong coloration, one arrives at $x = \frac{1}{458}$ and $n = \frac{1}{460'}$ for $\alpha = 860$ miles in the second. – As a result of the above, the rays contained in retreating white light change to those of a longer vibration time, such as violet to blue, blue through green to yellow, yellow through orange to red, and the red finally becoming completely extinguished through the increasing speed, i.e., they are no longer perceived. In the reverse case, where the blue rays disappear at first, the white light first appears to be green, then blue and finally violet. –

§ 6

All that has been said about the infuence of motion on light can be conveniently summarised in the following points:

1. If a glowing object, regardless of whether it is radiating the light itself or if it is merely illuminated by another source, is moving directly towards or away from the human eye with a speed comparable to the speed of light, this movement necessarily results in a change of the colour and intensity of the light, as follows:
   - α. When approaching, the intensity increases; the coloration, however, changes with increasing speed from white to green, from there to blue and finally to violet.
   - β. When retreating, the intensity weakens in all cases and the white light gradually turns to yellow, orange and lastly to red. If the light already has a certain coloration, e.g., a yellow one, the changes start from here and move up or down according to the conditions set out in α and β.

γ. Ist die Geschwindigkeit gross genug, so kann in beiden Fällen das weisse oder farbige Licht völlig insensibel werden, indem im ersteren Falle die Zeitintervalle der einzelnen Pulsationen zu klein, im zweiten dagegen zu gross ausfallen, um noch empfunden werden zu können. Die Intensität nimmt mit der Farbänderung übereinstimmend zu und ab, und trägt somit noch dazu bei, dass der genannte Erfolg des völligen Verschwindens bedeutend früher eintritt.

δ. Zum völligen Verschwinden eines im weissen Lichte glänzenden Gestirnes reicht ohne Rücksichtsnahme auf die diesem Ereignisse sehr günstige Intensitätsverminderung eine Geschwindigkeit von 19000 Meilen in der Sekunde hin. Für Sterne, die im homogenen gelben oder rothen Lichte leuchten, ist dagegen schon eine Geschwindigkeit von beziehungsweise 5007 und 1700 Meilen zum völligen Verlöschen ausreichend.

ε. Sterne, die im weissen Lichte leuchten, zeigen schon bei einer Geschwindigkeit von 33 Meilen in der Sekunde eine deutliche Färbung, und bei einer solchen von 187 Meilen eine sehr bedeutende und auffallende, die jedoch noch immer mit vielen weissen Strahlen vermischt ist. —

ϛ. Aendert sich die Geschwindigkeit eines bewegten Sternes, so erleidet auch seine Farbe und Intensität eine Aenderung, und so kann es immerhin geschehen, dass ein Stern im Verlaufe der Zeit alle Farben des Spectrums uns zu durchlaufen scheint.

2. Ist dagegen das leuchtende Object in Ruhe, der Beobachter dagegen in einer direct gegen oder von demselben gerichteten, bedeutend schnellen Bewegung begriffen, so erfolgen zwar alle Veränderungen in demselben Sinne, d. h. entsprechend der Annäherung oder dem Entfernen, die numerischen Daten jedoch weichen von jenen, den unter 1 und 2 aufgeführten Fällen entsprechenden Bestimmungen mehr oder weniger ab.

3. Geschieht das Annähern oder das sich Entfernen nicht wie es in 1 und 2 vorausgesetzt wird, directe, d. h. in der Richtung ihrer anfänglichen Verbindungslinie, sondern geht es in einer Richtung vor sich, die mit jener einen Winkel einschliesst; so ändert sich nebst der Farbe und Intensität auch noch die Richtung, und der Stern erleidet zugleich eine scheinbare Ortsveränderung.

Erkennt man die bisher aufgestellten Grundsätze für richtig an, so wird man gerne auch zugestehen, dass sie gleichsam die Grundlage einer neuen Theorie bilden, von welcher das berühmte Bradley'sche Aberrations-Theorem nur einen Theil vorstellet. Dem gemäss wird man sich schon a priori zu nachfolgenden Behauptungen für berechtiget halten dürfen. Wenn als die natürliche Farbe der Sterne die weisse oder schwachgelbliche angenommen wird, und es unter der unzählbaren Menge derselben solche gibt, die sich mit einer Geschwindigkeit von 33 Meilen bis zu 19000 Meilen in der Sekunde bewegen, so muss der gestirnte Himmel uns die Erscheinung einzelner Sterne jeder Farbe darbieten und es müssen einige von ihnen sogar zeitweilig ganz verschwinden, andere dagegen scheinbar entstehen; und umgekehrt, wenn uns eine genaue Beobachtung des Himmels wirklich solche Erscheinungen, wie sie so eben aufgezählt wurden, ganz unzweifelhaft zeiget, so liesse sich hieraus der Schluss ziehen, dass es unter den Gestirnen des Himmels einzelne Sterne geben dürfte, die sich mit einer

γ. If the speed is great enough, the white or coloured light can in both cases become totally imperceptible, in the first case by the time intervals between the pulsations becoming too small, and in the second case by becoming too large to be perceived. The intensity increases and decreases in harmony with the change in colour and therefore also contributes to the fact that the resulting total disappearance takes place significantly earlier.

δ. To making a shining white star disappear completely, all that is required, ignoring the favourable effect of the reduction in intensity, is a speed of 84 000 miles in the second. For stars which shine with homogeneous yellow or red light, a speed of 23 000 and 7 830 miles respectively is sufficient to result in complete extinction.

ε. Stars that shine with a white light, already show at a speed of 152 miles in the second a distinctive coloration which becomes at 860 miles even more significant and noticable, but it is still mixed with many white rays. –

φ. If the speed of a moving star changes, its colour and intensity also undergo a change and so it can happen that a star appears to range through all the colours of the spectrum in the course of time.

2. If, on the other hand, the shining object is stationary and it is the observer who is subjected to significantly rapid motion directly towards or away from the aforementioned, there will be changes in the same way, i.e., as far as the movements together or apart are concerned, but the numerical data, however, differ to a greater or lesser extent from those conditions given in the cases under 1.

3. If the approaching or distancing does not take place directly, as is the case in 1 and 2, i.e., following the path of their original connecting line, but moves off at an angle, then not only the colour and intensity change but also the direction and the star undergoes at the same time an apparent change of location.

If one accepts these principles as being correct, one will also admit that they form the basis of a new theory of which *Bradley's* famous aberration theorum forms only a part. Accordingly, one will already *a priori* hold the following claims as justified. If it is accepted that the natural colour of the stars is white or a weak yellow, and there are among the innumerable amounts of these, those which move at speeds between 152 miles and 84 000 miles in the second, so must the starry sky present us individual stars in various colours and a few of them must even temporarily disappear whereas others appear newly-created; and conversely, if a close observation of the sky really shows such appearances as just described, the conclusion must be made among the constellations of the heavens

Geschwindigkeit von 33 Meilen bis 19000 Meilen im Weltraume bewegen. Wenn aber endlich nicht nur die erwähnten Erscheinungen am Himmel mit Gewissheit beobachtet, sondern es auch durch genaue Beobachtungen und aus mechanischen Gründen als erwiesen anzusehen wäre, dass einige dieser Himmelskörper wirklich eine Geschwindigkeit von 33 bis 19000 Meilen besitzen, ja noch überdiess, dass gerade eben nur an diesen schnellbewegten Körpern nach Massgabe der oben aufgestellten Grundsätze sich jene Farben- und Intensitäts-Erscheinungen zeigen: so würde dieses hinwieder für die Richtigkeit der hier aufgestellten Theorie und weiter zurück sogar für das Stattfinden der Longitudinal-Schwingungen ein sehr beachtenswerthes und gewichtiges Zeugniss ablegen. — Unter diesen Umständen fühlt man sich aufgefordert, sich nach den Angaben der beobachtenden Astronomie umzusehen. —

§. 7.

Bekanntlich ist es bisher den Bemühungen der Astronomen und Physiker noch keineswegs gelungen, die höchst merkwürdige und wahrhaft räthselhafte Erscheinung der mit farbigem Lichte leuchtenden sogenannten Doppelsterne und einiger anderer Gestirne des Himmels auf eine auch nur halbwegs befriedigende Weise zu erklären. An und für sich und im ersten Augenblicke mag es wohl scheinen, als hätte man um so weniger einen Grund, sich über farbige Fixsterne im Allgemeinen zu wundern, als sich ja auch auf unserer Erde selbst und im Bereiche der täglichen Erfahrung leuchtende Körper jeder Farbe genug vorfinden. Allein eine genauere Erwägung aller dabei obwaltenden Umstände muss wohl jeden von dieser anfänglichen Meinung, falls er sie gefasst, gar bald wieder zurückbringen. Denn abgesehen selbst von anderem, muss es schon in hohem Grade auffallen, dass wir nnter der unzählbaren Menge der eigentlichen, d. i. derjenigen Fixsterne, an denen wir keinerlei Bewegung wahrnehmen, ohne Ausnahme nur solche bemerken, die im weissen oder schwach gelblichen und nur einige wenige, die im röthlichen Lichte glänzen; keinen einzigen dagegen, welcher im blauen, grünen oder violetten und keinen auch der im schön orangen oder intensiv blutrothen Lichte uns erschiene. Alle Doppelsterne dagegen lassen sich übersichtlich in zwei Classen bringen, in solche, bei denen der eine von ihnen sich durch seine in die Augen fallende grössere Intensität seines Lichtes als Haupt- oder Centralstern beurkundet, und sodann in solche, deren Einzelnsterne eine ziemlich gleiche scheinbare Grösse besitzen, und die sich daher auch höchst wahrscheinlich um einen unsichtbaren Centralkörper oder um ihren gemeinschaftlichen Schwerpunkt bewegen. — Bei den Doppelsternen der ersteren Art leuchtet der Hauptstern stets im weissen und nur bei wenigen im schwach gelblichen Lichte, und zeiget somit eine vollkommene Übereinstimmung mit den übrigen unbeweglichen Fixsternen des Himmels, während dagegen die dazu gehörigen Begleiter entweder im grünen, blauen oder violetten, bei andern dagegen im intensiv orangen, schön blut- oder wohl auch dunkelrothen Lichte glänzen. — Doppelsterne der zweiten Classe bestehen dagegen fast immer aus solchen Einzelnsternen, die im verschiedenfarbigen Lichte schimmern, und merkwürdig ist es dabei, dass die Farben entweder wirklich einen complementären Gegensatz zu einander bilden, oder dass wenigstens die Farbe des einen dem obern, die des andern dem untern Theile des Farben-

there must be some stars that move in space with a speed 152 to 84 000 miles. When it is finally possible not only to make observations of these appearances with certainty, but by a more exact study and on mechanical grounds to prove that some of these heavenly bodies truly have a speed between 152 and 84 000 miles, and furthermore that only these fast travelling bodies comply with the changes in colour and intensity referred to above, so would this be respected and weighty evidence for the theory put forward here and the existence of longitudinal oscillations. – Under these circumstances one feels challenged to consider this information in respect to observational astronomy.

§ 7

As is well known, the efforts until now of astronomers and physicists to even halfway explain the strange and truly puzzling appearance of the so-called double stars which radiate coloured light, and certain other stars of the heavens, have remained fruitless. At the first glance it might appear that there is little reason to wonder about the coloured stars altogether, since there are here on our Earth and in our daily lives enough glowing objects of every colour. Only a closer consideration of the above circumstances must convince anyone who was of the previous opinion soon to change his mind. Above other things it must seem patently obvious that, among the innumerable masses of fixed stars in which we can see no movement whatsoever, there are, without exception, only those that shine with a white or weak yellow or in a very few cases, a reddish light; not a single one, on the other hand, which appears to us as blue, green or violet, and also none that shine with a beautiful orange or intense blood red. All the double stars, however, can be conveniently brought into two classes: in those which, because of the greater intensity falling on the eye can thus be designated as the main or central star, and in those where the single stars are of seemingly equal size and are therefore most probably moving around an invisible central body or their common centre of gravity. – With the double stars of the first type it is the main star that shines with a white or with a few cases a weak yellow light, and shows therefore a complete harmony with the rest of the stationary fixed stars in the sky. The accompanying stars which belong to them are, on the other hand, either green, blue or violet, whilst others shine with an intense orange, beautiful blood red or even dark red. – Double stars of the second class nearly always consist of stars which shine in different coloured light and the strange

2*

spectrums entnommen ist. Man hat zwar versucht, wiewohl mit wenig Glück, die genannten Erscheinungen aus den Wirkungen des Contrastes zu erklären. Allein abgesehen davon, dass diese Erklärung im günstigsten Falle höchstens nur auf jene Doppelsterne angewendet werden könnte, bei denen das vorkommende farbige Licht in einem complementären, nicht aber in einem andern Gegensatze sich befindet, wie dieses doch bei allen der ersten und bei sehr vielen der zweiten Classe der Fall ist, — haben noch überdiess directe Versuche das Unhaltbare dieser Ansicht seither zur Genüge dargethan. Diese Versuche bestanden bekanntlich darin, dass man den einen der farbigen Doppelsterne durch einen im Fernrohre ausgespannten Faden völlig verdeckte und somit dem Auge gänzlich entzog. Da nun hiedurch die angebliche Ursache des Contrastes wegfiel, so hätte auch die Wirkung davon, nämlich das Erscheinen der complementären Farbe ausbleiben sollen. Dieses aber geschah nicht und der Stern leuchtete vor wie nach mit demselben farbigen Lichte. — Damit das Mass des Wunderbaren endlich voll werde, hat eine Vergleichung der älteren Angaben *Herschels* d. ä. mit den neuesten *Struve's* noch überdiess bis zur Evidenz es herausgestellt, dass die Farben vieler dieser Doppelsterne im Verlaufe dieser Zeit sich sehr bedeutend und zwar auf eine Weise geändert haben, die der Vermuthung keinen Raum gewährt, als wäre der Grund dieser Verschiedenheit in der Beschaffenheit der hier und dort angewandten optischen Instrumente zu suchen. Sterne, die ehemals als gelb beobachtet wurden, werden heut zu Tage als orange und roth und umgekehrt beschrieben und solche, die *Herschel* als vollkommen weiss bezeichnet, findet *Struve* goldfarbig, rothgrün oder auch blaugrün! — Kein Wunder also, wenn sich neuere Beobachter (siehe *Mädlers* pop. Astronomie, S. 493) zu der Frage aufgefordert fühlen, »ob sich denn in der That die Farben der Doppelsterne während der letzten 50 Jahre so gar bedeutend sollten geändert haben?«

§. 8.

Eine andere, nicht minder interessante und bisher ebenso unaufgeklärte Erscheinung des Himmels sind die sogenannten periodisch veränderlichen Sterne. Sie kommen nach den bisherigen Beobachtungen mit alleiniger Ausnahme des Sternes Algol im Medusenhaupte (von dem später noch die Rede seyn wird) insgesammt darin überein, dass sie von Farbe roth sind, nach ihrem grössten Glanze eine Kupferfarbe annehmen, und indem diese allmählig sich mehr und mehr verdunkelt, endlich völlig unsichtbar werden und verschwinden, bis sie nach einiger Zeit ihren periodischen Lichtwechsel wieder von vorne beginnen. Auch darin kommen sie ferner miteinander überein, dass die Zeit ihrer Unsichtbarkeit meistentheils 3- bis 4mal länger währt, als jene ihres grössten Glanzes, und endlich, dass ihre Lichtzunahme viel rascher vor sich gehet und weniger Zeit erfordert, wie ihre Abnahme und ihr Verschwinden. Die Art und Weise der Lichtzu- und Abnahme ist mit der Voraussetzung unverträglich, dass dieses zeitweilige Verschwinden in einer Achsendrehung und ungleichen Lichtvertheilung auf der Oberfläche dieser Himmelskörper, oder auch in einem periodischen Verdecktwerden durch einen umkreisenden dunkeln Planeten seinen Grund habe. — Auf den ersten Augenblick scheint es, als ob die beiden erwähnten, so verschiedenartigen Erscheinungen, nämlich jene

thing is that the colours are either truly complementary to each other, or at least the colour of one is from the upper part of the spectrum and the other from the lower part. It has been tried to explain this, but with little success, by the effects of contrast. Putting aside the fact that this explanation will at best only apply to those double stars whose coloured light is complementary but not of another opposing colour, as is the case in all of the first and many of the second class, – direct experiments have in addition shown this view to be untenable. These experiments consisted of looking at the double stars through a telescope in which a thread was strung in such a way that it completely covered one of the stars. Since in this way the apparent origin of the contrast was eliminated, its effect, namely the appearance of the complementary colour, should have disappeared. This did not happen and the star kept on shining with the same coloured light as before. In order that the cup of wonders should be filled to the brim, a comparison of the older data of *Herschel* the elder with the newer ones of *Stuve* have made it evident that the colours of many of these double stars have changed significantly during the course of time, and in such a way as to eliminate all speculation that these differences could be attributable to the characteristics of the optical instruments used here and there. Stars that had previously been observed as being yellow are now being described as being red or orange, and vice versa, and those that *Herschel* designated as completely white, *Struve* finds to be golden, red-green or blue-green! No wonder therefore that the new observers (see *Mädler's* Pop. Astronomy, p. 439) feel obliged to ask "if in reality the colours of the double stars have changed so significantly during the last 50 years?"

§ 8

Another not less interesting and hitherto unexplained phenomenon of the heavens are the so-called periodically changing stars. With the exception of the star Algol at the head of Medusa (of whom there will be more later) they have in common that they are red in colour, after their brightest moment they take on a copper colour which becomes darker and darker until the star has become invisible, and vanish, until some time they start their periodic change of light all over again. Another characteristic they have in common is that the time of their invisibility is mostly 3 to 4 times longer than that of their brightest time, and lastly, the time that it takes for their light to increase is much less than the time for the dimming and disappearing. The nature of the light increase and decrease is not compatible with the assumption that the periodic disappearance is due to an axial turn and uneven light distribution, or even a periodic cover from a circling dark planet. – At the first glance it seems as if both

der farbigen Doppelsterne und die der sogenannten veränderlichen Sterne, nur mit einigem Zwange ein und demselben Erklärungsprincipe untergeordnet werden könnten. Allein die Beobachtung hat uns noch mit einer dritten Classe von merkwürdigen Sternveränderungen bekannt gemacht, die gleichsam zwischen beiden mitten innestehen und als wahre Vermittlungsglieder dieser Erscheinungsgruppen betrachtet werden können. Es sind dieses die verschwundenen und neuen Sterne.

Hieher nun gehört vorzüglich der im Jahre 1572 im Sternbilde der Cassiopeia erschienene neue Stern, welchem man eine Umlaufszeit oder Periodicität seines Lichtwechsels von etwa 300, vielleicht gar nur von 150 Jahren beilegen zu müssen glaubt. Als man auf ihn aufmerksam wurde, hatte er bereits nahe schon das Maximum seiner scheinbaren Grösse und der Intensität seines Lichtes erreicht und überstrahlte mit blendend weissem Lichte den Sirius und selbst die Venus. Bald darauf nahm er an Grösse schnell ab und sein Licht ging gleichzeitig und allmählig von Weiss in Gelb und von diesem in Roth über, welches immer dunkler wurde und endlich für die Beobachtung ganz erlosch. (*Richter's* Astronomie, S. 684.) — Noch auffallender waren die Erscheinungen bei dem im Jahre 1604 von *Kepler* im Fusse des Schlangenträgers entdeckten neuen Stern. Nachdem sein Licht durch alle Farben des Regenbogens niedersteigend abgenommen hatte, verschwand er nach etwa einem Jahre und ist seitdem niemals wieder gesehen worden. Endlich erwähnen auch Schriftsteller früherer Zeiten ähnlicher Erscheinungen, und vom Sirius, der gegenwärtig in blendend weissem Lichte strahlt, soll es keinem Zweifel unterliegen, dass er ehemals ein rothes Licht hatte u. a. m. — Es haben demnach diese Gestirne mit den Doppelsternen das Farbenspiel und mit grosser Wahrscheinlichkeit die schnelle Bewegung, so wie die meistentheils auf Jahrhunderte sich erstreckende lange Periodicität, — mit den sogenannten veränderlichen Sternen dagegen das völlige Verschwinden und gänzliche Unsichtbarwerden, so wie auch, dass sie ungleich länger unsichtbar wie sichtbar sind, und endlich, dass die Lichtabnahme von längerer Dauer ist, wie die Lichtzunahme und noch mehreres andere gemein. — Wir sehen daher alle diejenigen Erscheinungen an den verschiedenen Objecten des Himmels wirklich durch Beobachtungen nachgewiesen, die wir oben unter Voraussetzung einer ihnen zukommenden grossen Geschwindigkeit ihrer Bewegung bis ins Detail prognostizirten. Wir wollen uns daher noch weiter umsehen, was die unmittelbare Beobachtung und Berechnung, wie auch die Wahrscheinlichkeit uns rücksichtlich ihrer Bewegung selbst lehrt. —

§. 9.

Die Geschwindigkeit der Planeten unseres Sonnensystems, selbst wenn sie sich im Perihelio befinden, ist vergleichungsweise noch nicht sehr bedeutend. Die Erde bewegt sich mit einer Geschwindigkeit von beiläufig 4·7 Meilen, bei der Venus beträgt sie 6·7 und beim Merkur 8·3 Meilen in der Sekunde. Kein Wunder also, dass wir an ihnen bisher noch keine Farbenänderung und noch weniger ein zeitweiliges völliges Verschwinden beobachtet haben. Wäre die Geschwindigkeit unserer Erde wenigstens zehnmal so gross als sie wirklich ist, so müssten uns alle Fixsterne in den östlichen Gegenden der Ecliptik ohne Ausnahme mit blauer

of the very different appearances mentioned, namely that of the coloured double stars and that of the so-called variable stars, can only be placed into the same explanatory principle. Simple observation has familiarised us with a third class of strange changes in stars which stand equally between both and can be seen as the true explanatory link in these groups of phenomena. They are those of the lost and the new stars.

An excellent example here is the new star which appeared in 1572 under the stellar sign of Cassiopeia, whose periodicity of light change was believed to be 300, perhaps only 150 years. When it was first noticed, it was close to reaching what seemed to be its maximum size and intensity, and with ts bright white light it outshone Sirius and even Venus. Soon thereafter it diminished in size and its light gradually changed from white to yellow and then to red, which became darker and darker and then completely disappeared from observation *(Richter's* Astronomy, p. 684). – Even more noticeable were the appearances of the new star found in the year 1604 at the foot of Ophiuchus the Snakebearer by *Keppler.* After its light passed diminishingly down through all the colours of the rainbow, it vanished after about a year and has not been seen since. Lastly, writers of earlier times mention similar phenomena, and Sirius, which is at present emitting a dazzling white light, without any doubt once emitted a red light, and so on. – Therefore these stars have this play of light in common with the double stars and most probably the high speed, as well as their long periodicity which for the most part lasts centuries. – With the so-called changing stars, on the other hand, they share the fact that they disappear totally and become invisible, as well as that they are invisible unequally longer than visible, and finally, that the decrease of light is longer in duration than the increase, and much else in common. – We therefore see all those appearances of the various objects in the sky confirmed by observations, which are prognosed in detail above, on the basis of the high speed at which they travel. We therefore want to seek further afield and see what close observation and calculation, and also probability, teaches us about their movement itself. –

§ 9

The speed of the planets in our solar system, even if they are located in the perihelion, is in comparison not very significant. The Earth moves with a speed of approximately 21.6 miles, with Venus it is 30.8 and Mercury 38.2 miles in the second. No wonder therefore that until now we have seen no changes of colour or, even less, a temporary but complete disappearance of these. Were the speed of our Earth at least ten times as large as it really is, so would all all fixed stars in the eastern regions of

oder grünlicher Färbung, auf der entgegengesetzten westlichen Seite dagegen orange oder roth erscheinen. Durch eine so auffallende, auf alle Fixsterne in gleicher Weise sich erstreckende Regelmässigkeit eines solchen Phänomens aufmerksam gemacht, würde man, wie einstens bei jenem der Aberration, die Ursache davon in der Bewegung der Erde suchen und finden. So aber, wo diese Erscheinungen nur vereinzelnt auftreten, da' sie auch nur in den vorzugsweise schnellen Bewegungen einzelner Fixsterne ihren Grund haben, muss es schon viel schwieriger seyn, dieselben bis ins kleinste Detail zu erklären, und höchst wahrscheinlich gehören absichtlich zu diesem Zwecke veranstaltete Beobachtungsreihen dazu. — Die Monde bewegen sich bekanntlich bald langsamer, bald schneller wie ihre Planeten, und es mag dahin gestellt bleiben, ob nicht einige an ihnen wahrgenommene Eigenthümlichkeiten hieher zu zählen seyn dürften? — Viel bedeutender dagegen ist schon die an den Kometen beobachtete Geschwindigkeit ihrer Bewegung. Der *Halley'sche* Komet hat im Perihelio nahe 18 Meilen Geschwindigkeit in der Sekunde, und jener vom Jahre 1680 bewegte sich in der Sonnennähe mit einer Geschwindigkeit von 74 Meilen in der Sekunde und somit nahe 17mal so geschwind wie unsere Erde. Es ist gar nicht daran zu zweifeln, dass es selbst schon unter den bisher beobachteten aber nicht berechneten Kometen früherer Zeit einen oder den andern gegeben haben mag, dessen Geschwindigkeit mehre hundert Meilen in der Sekunde erreichte. Bei diesen nun ist eine schwache Färbung in Folge ihrer schnellen Bewegung nicht unwahrscheinlich, und soll auch wirklich bei einigen derselben beobachtet worden seyn. Dass es hierbei auf die Richtung ihrer Bewegung und auf die Lage ihrer Bahnen gegen unsere Erde ankömmt, versteht sich fast von selbst, und es wäre interessant, die damalige Stellung unserer Erde gegen die Bahnen jener Komaten wo möglich zu ermitteln. Dadurch aber, dass wir unserer Erde die Fähigkeit absprechen, für sich allein merkbare Farb- und Intensitätsänderungen an den verschiedenen Himmelskörpern in Folge ihrer fortschreitenden Bewegung zu bewirken, wollen wir keineswegs zugleich behaupten, dass dieselbe nicht auf das frühere oder spätere Eintreffen jener Erscheinungen und auf den Grad derselben einen sehr merkbaren Einfluss ausüben werde, ja sogar nothwendigerweise ausüben müsse. Höchst wahrscheinlich haben einige an den periodisch veränderlichen Sternen beobachtete Anomalien, von denen weiter unten noch die Rede seyn wird, hierin ihren erklärenden Grund. — In Betreff der Fixsterne ermangelt es eines jeden Grundes, anzunehmen, dass unsere Sonne sie alle insgesammt an Masse und Grösse übertreffe. Es kann vielmehr für eine stehende Ansicht in der Astronomie gelten, dass es höchst wahrscheinlich Fixsterne geben dürfte, welche unsere Sonne im Durchmesser, um vielleicht mehrere Hundertmal, an Masse sie um eben so viele Millionenmal übertreffen mögen. Nun hängt aber die Geschwindigkeit mit welcher sich Satelliten um ihre Centralkörper bewegen, unter gleichen Umständen direct von der Masse desselben ab, und man hätte daher unter so bewandten Umständen keinen Grund, sich sehr darüber zu wundern, wenn uns die Beobachtung wirklich an einigen dieser Himmelskörper Bewegungen zeigte, deren Geschwindigkeit selbst die des Lichtes übertreffen. In der That hat man an den sogenannten Doppelsternen und höchst wahrsaheinlish auch an den veränderlichen und neuen Sternen derlei schnell bewegte Gestirne kennen gelernt. Ich begnüge

the ecliptic appear without exception in a blue or greenish coloration, whereas on the opposite western side they must appear orange or red. Having been made aware of such a regularity which uniformly spans the phenonenon of all fixed stars, one would, as one did earlier with that of aberration, search for the reason in the movement of the Earth and find it there. But where these phenomena appear only sporadically, since their existence lies in a favourably rapid movement of just a few fixed stars, it is far more difficult to explain these down to the last detail, and most probably a series of observations would have to be carried out for this purpose. – As is known, the moons move sometimes faster, sometimes slower than their planets and it might be asked if some of the characteristics they display should not be reckoned with here? – Much more important though is the speed that has been observed in the movement of comets. *Halley's* comet has in the perihelion a speed of almost 38 miles in the second, and the one of 1680 moved in the vicinity of the Sun with a speed of 340 miles in the second, and thus almost 17 times the speed of our Earth. It is not to be doubted that already among the previously observed but not calculated comets of earlier times, there was one or the other whose speed reached a few hundred miles in the second. With these, a weak coloration as a result of their rapid motion is not unlikely, and has actually been observed in some of them. That the direction of their movement and the relation of their paths to our Earth play a great role is obvious, and it would be interesting to determine the location of our Earth at that time in relation to the paths of those comets. However, because we deny our Earth's ability to cause on its own noticable changes in colour and intensity in the various heavenly bodies through continuously increasing speed, we by no means claim at the same time that this may not exert a very noticable influence – yes, even must necessarily exert such an influence – on earlier or later arrival of such appearances and on the degree of the same. Most probably, some anomalies which have been observed in the periodically changing stars, and which will be mentioned again below, can be explained in this way. – Concerning the fixed stars, there is no reason to presume that our Sun exceeds them all in size and mass. It can rather be regarded as an established astronomical viewpoint that there are likely to be fixed stars which exceed the radius of the Sun by a few hundred times, its mass by many millions. However, the speed with which a satellite moves around its central body depends, under equal circumstances, directly upon the mass of the same, and there is, therefore, no reason to marvel too much when observation shows us in reality that some of these heavenly bodies move with speeds in excess of that of light itself. In fact, with the so-called double stars, and most likely also with the variable and new stars, one has learned of

mich dasjenige anzuführen, was ein geachteter Astronom (siehe *Littrow's* W. d. H. S. 470) rüchsichtlich des Doppelsterns γ in der Jungfrau berichtet. „Merkwürdig," sagt er, »ist die grosse Geschwindigkeit dieses Satelliten zur Zeit seines Periheliums, wo er in einem Tage einen Weg von 3190 Millionen Meilen und somit in einer Sekunde nahe an 40,000 Meilen zurücklegt, und somit fast genau ebenso schnell sich bewegt, wie das Licht selbst.« Mag man daher immerhin in diesem speciellen Falle diesen mehr auf einer ungefähren Schätzung als auf genauen Beobachtungen beruhenden Angaben keinen grossen Grad von Genauigkeit zuschreiben: so geht doch jedenfalls aus selben so viel hervor, dass die Annahme einer Geschwindigkeit von 33 bis 19000 Meilen in der Sekunde, mit welcher ein oder der andere der Fixsterne sich bewegen mag, weder für unwahrscheinlich, noch für im mindesten übertrieben zu halten ist.

§. 10.

Es ist gewiss im höchsten Grade auffallend, dass wir gerade nur an jenen Himmelskörpern so bedeutende Veränderungen in Farbe und Intensität des Lichtes wahrnehmen, bei denen wir entweder zufolge unmittelbarer Beobachtung eine ganz ausserordentlich grosse Geschwindigkeit ihrer Bewegung vorauszusetzen berechtigt sind, oder aber, bei welchen wir diese vermöge aller Analogie voraussetzen können, während bei allen übrigen Gestirnen des Himmels, die wir vergleichungsweise für ruhende oder wenigstens für viel minder schnell sich bewegende anzunehmen genöthigt sind, solche Erscheinungen ohne Ausnahme nicht vorkommen. Man fühlt sich daher sehr zu der Meinung hingezogen, dass sämmtliche Gestirne des Himmels an und für sich im weissen oder schwach gelblichen Lichte schimmern, und dass, wenn dieses bei einzelnen anders gefunden wird, ein Grund dafür bestehen müsse, welcher mit der grossen Geschwindigkeit ihrer Bewegung höchst wahrscheinlich in einem nicht bloss zufälligen, sondern nothwendigen Zusammenhange steht. Es war der Zweck der gegenwärtigen Abhandlung, nicht etwa bloss die allenfallsige Möglichkeit, sondern die Nothwendigkeit eines solchen Einflusses der ungemein schnellen Bewegung der Himmelskörper auf ihre Farbe und auf die Intensität ihres Lichtes darzuthun, und es gewährt dem Verfasser derselben eine erfreuliche Genugthuung, die vollkommenste Uebereinstimmung der Beobachtungen, insoweit sie ihm bekannt sind, mit den oben aufgestellten Grundsätzen oft selbst bis ins Detail wahrzunehmen. Es möge daher gestattet seyn, auf einige derselben hier aufmerksam zu machen. Es erklärt sich hieraus ganz einfach:

1. Warum von den beiden Doppelsternen der grössere und somit wahrscheinlich beziehungsweise unbewegliche Central- oder Hauptstern fast ausnahmslos weiss, der beigegebene dagegen meistentheils farbig erscheint!
2. Warum in jenen Fällen, wo beide ziemlich gleich gross erscheinen, beide gefärbt sich zeigen!
3. Wesshalb in diesem letztern Falle der eine fast immer mit einem Lichte glänzt, welches dem obern Theile des Farbenspectrums zugehört (also grün, blau, violet), der zugehörige dagegen mit einer Farbe aus dem untern Theile desselben (also roth, orange oder gelb)

such fast-moving stars. It suffices to state what a respected astronomer (see *Littrow's* Wonder of the Heavens, p. 470) has reported concerning the double star γ in Virgo. “Strange,” he says, “is the great speed of this satellite at the time of its perihelium, when in one day it covers 16 000 million miles, and thus in a second nearly 186 000 miles, and thus travelling almost as fast as the light itself.” – One may, though, not give too great a degree of accuracy to this special case, which is based more on an approximate estimate than on exact observations: yet, from it can be seen that the acceptance of a speed from 152 to 84 000 miles in the second with which one or the other fixed star might travel, is neither to be regarded as unrealistic nor in the slightest exaggerated.

§ 10

It is to a great extent obvious that we only perceive in heavenly bodies those important changes in colour and intensity where either direct observation entitles us to presume a very exceptional great speed, or those in which this can be presumed on the strength of all analogy, whereas with all other stars of the sky that we see as being stationary, or at least as being very much slower in comparison, have without exception not displayed such appearances. One feels therefore drawn to the opinion that all of the stars of the sky shine with either white or a weak yellow light, and if some are found to be different then there must be a reason, which most likely stands in a not merely coincidental relationship to the great speed of their movement. It was the purpose of this present discourse to show not merely the vague possibility, but the necessity of such an influence from the enormously fast speeds of the heavenly bodies on the colour and intensity of their light, and the author of the above has derived a great deal of satisfaction in seeing that all observations known to him are in complete accordance with the principles set out above, often down to the last detail. It may be allowed, therefore, to draw attention to some of these. It is to be explained from this quite simply:

1. Why from both double stars the larger, and therewith probably the stationary central or main star is almost without exception white, whereas the partner star mostly appears coloured!
2. Why, in those cases where both appear of approximately equal size, both are coloured!
3. Why in this last case that one shines with a light which belongs to the upper part of the colour spectrum (green, blue, violet) the partner on the other hand with a colour from the lower part

Denn bei gleichgrossen Doppelsternen kann füglich angenommen werden, insbesondere, wenn sie sich um ihren gemeinschaftlichen Schwerpunkt bewegen, dass der eine in der Annäherung begriffen ist, während sich der andere von uns entfernt.

4. Es erklärt sich hieraus äusserst einfach, warum die Farben der einzelnen Doppelsterne mit der Zeit sich so bedeutend ändern. So z. B. bezeichnet *Herschel* d. ält. den schönsten Doppelstern des Nordens, nämlich γ Leonis, den einen schön weiss und den dazu gehörigen weissröthlich, während *Struve* den Hauptstern goldfarbig und den Nebenstern rothgrün findet. Noch auffallender ist dieses bei dem Doppelstern γ Delphini. Bei den so auffallenden und deutlichen Farben, goldgelb und blaugrün (sagt *Mädler*, p. Astronomie, S. 500) ist es sehr zu verwundern, dass sie *Herschel* ausdrücklich beide weiss nennt. — Wir aber müssen zufolge unsers Erklärungsprincipes noch hinzufügen, dass eine Zeit kommen wird, wo diese Doppelsterne sogar dieses ihr farbiges Licht wechselseitig austauschen werden. Die Doppelsterne durchlaufen also während jeder ihrer Revolutionsperioden die Farbenscala des Sonnenspectrums, zum wenigsten einen Theil derselben.

5. Es erklärt sich hieraus ferner das merkwürdige Verhalten der periodisch veränderlichen Sterne, und warum namentlich die Farbe dieser Sterne gerade die rothe ist. Denn entweder sind sie an und für sich für uns unsichtbare Sterne (vielleicht wegen zu geringer Intensität oder zu langer Schwingungsdauer), die nur durch ihre gegen uns gerichtete schnelle Bewegung die erste Stufe der Wahrnehmbarkeit erreichen, d. h. uns mit rothem Lichte erscheinen. Vielleicht aber sind sie in der That von röthlichem Lichte und verschwinden uns in Folge der von uns weggerichteten Beweguug.

6. Auch noch der Umstand der kurzen Zeit ihres Sichtbarseyns im Vergleiche zu ihrer Periodicität findet durch den Hinblick auf Fig. 5 und 6 eine genügende Erklärung, ja folgt gewissermassen mit Nothwendigkeit aus derselben. Dem ungefähr während voller drei Viertel seines Umlaufs und oft viel mehr noch, je nach der Lage und Form der Ellipse gegen den Beobachter, muss ein solcher nur durch sein Annähern, also immer nur während der Zeit seines Periheliums uns sichtbar gewordener Stern uns unsichtbar bleiben. Diess tritt besonders auffallend hervor, wenn man als Bahn eine Ellipse von bedeutender Excentricität und von einer Lage gegen den Beobachter voraussetzt, wie die in Fig. 6 dargestellte ist.

7. Die früher erwähnte Erscheinung, dass die veränderlichen Sterne meistentheils eine viel kürzere Zeit zur Zunahme als zur Abnahme des Lichtes bedürfen, findet gleichfalls in Fig. 7 eine genügende Erklärung. Bis kurz vor dem Eintritt ins Perihelium hat der Stern bei schon sehr bedeutender absoluter Geschwindigkeit noch eine so ungünstige Richtung seiner Bewegung, dass sich derselbe dem Beobachter in O gar nicht oder nur sehr wenig annähert, bis er in m angelangt, plötzlich in die günstigste Richtung, bei nahe noch grösster absoluter Geschwindigkeit, deren er fähig ist, eintritt. Noch günstiger für das Eintreffen dieses Ereignisses ist eine beziehungsweise Lage, wie jene in Fig. 8 vorgestellte, und man begreift demnach leicht, wie Sterne innerhalb weniger Stunden

of the same (red, orange or yellow). Then with equally large double stars it can justifiably be assumed, especially when they are moving around their common centre of gravity, that one approaches while the other is retreating from us.

4. It is explained from this, extremely simply, why the colours of the individual double stars change so significantly in the course of time. For example, *Herschel* the elder describes the most beautiful double star of the North, namely γ Leonis, the one as beautiful white and that belonging to it as white-reddish, while *Struve* finds the main star gold-coloured and the secondary star red-green. This is even more noticable with the double star γ Delphini. With such noticable and clear colours as golden yellow and bluish green (says *Mädler*, Popular Astronomy, p. 500) it is very surprising that *Herschel* expressly refers to them both as being white. – We must add as a result of the explanation of our principle that the time will even come when these two stars will exchange their coloured light. Thus the double stars, during their periodic revolution, run through the colour scale of the Sun's spectrum, or at least part of it.
5. It is further explained from this why the periodically changing stars behave so strangely and why the colour of these stars is just the red. Then they are, properly speaking, stars which are invisible for us (perhaps due to a too feeble intensity or a too long wavelength) which reach the first stage of perception only through their rapid speed in our direction, i.e., appear to us with red light. It may be, however, that they are of reddish light and disappear from us the result of their movement away from us.

Fig. 5
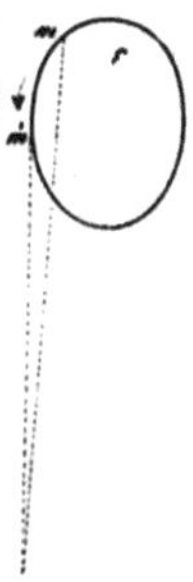

Fig. 6
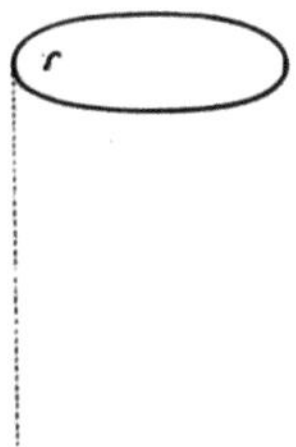

Fig. 7
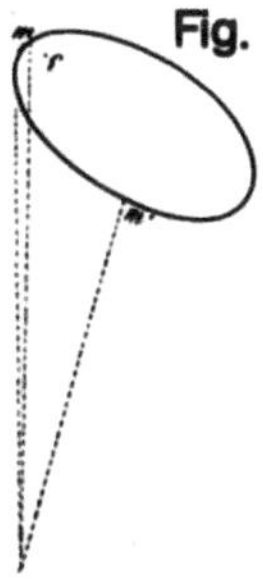

6. Also the circumstances of the short time of their visibility in comparison to their periodicity is satisfactorily explained in Figs. 5 and 6, and is, in a manner of speaking, its logical conclusion. During about a full three-quarters of its orbit, and often more depending upon the position and shape of the ellipse in relation to the observer, such a star must become visible to us only during its approach and thus remain invisible during its perihelion. This becomes very obvious if one has an elliptical orbit of significant eccentricity and position relative to the observer as shown in Fig. 6.
7. The phenomenon mentioned earlier, whereby the variable stars for the most part need a much shorter time to gain light than to lose it, finds an adequate explanation in Fig. 7 as well. Until shortly before its entry into the perihelion this star has, despite an already very significant absolute speed, such an unfavourable direction of movement that it approaches the observer at *O* very little or not at all until it reaches *m*, suddenly in the most favourable direction with almost greater absolute speed that it is capable of. Even more favourable for the occurance of this happening is the position shown in Fig. 8 and one can easily grasp from this how stars within a few

plötzlich sichtbar werden und dieses durch einige Zeit verbleiben, dann aber allmählig abnehmen und nach einigen Jahren völlig wieder verschwinden konnten.

8. Ebenso erklärt sich auch daraus, warum die sogenannten neuen und verschwundenen Sterne alle Farben des Regenbogens durchlaufend mit kupferrothem Lichte endlich verschwinden. Höchst wahrscheinlich dürfte keine geringe Anzahl derjenigen Sterne, die wir gewöhnlich für unbeweglich und unveränderlich halten, einem ähnlichen Farben- und Lichtwechsel unterworfen seyn, wie ja dieses in Bezug auf Sirius ausser Zweifel gestellt scheint.

9. Endlich dürften sich höchst wahrscheinlich die bei verschiedenen periodisch veränderlichen Sternen wahrgenommenen Anomalien aus der Bewegung unserer Erde erklären lassen. So z. B. zeigt der Stern Mira am Halse des Wallfisches bald eine Periode des Lichtwechsels von $328\frac{1}{2}$ Tagen, bald wieder eine von $335\frac{1}{2}$ Tagen, also einen Unterschied von 7 Tagen. Da nun die Umlaufszeit unserer Erde $365\frac{1}{4}$ Tage währt, so befindet sich die Erde zur Zeit, wo jener Stern zu seinem grössten Glanze gelangt, in jedem Jahre in einem andern Zeichen und die Richtung ihrer Bewegung gegen oder von jenem Sterne ist somit in verschiedenen Jahren eine verschiedene. Aber da die Bewegung der Erde auf das Eintreten in die Phase ihres grössten Glanzes ganz unzweifelhaft einen Einfluss ausüben muss, so wird dieselbe das einemal um etwas früher, das anderemal um eben so viel später erfolgen. Eine Geschwindigkeitsdifferenz von 9·4 Meilen würde daher das Verschwinden oder die Erlangung des grössten Glanzes um volle 7 Tage verzögern oder beschleunigen. Ist diess richtig, so müsste sich beim Stern Mira eine Periodicität dieser scheinbaren Anomalie von beiläufig 12 Jahren nachweisen lassen, und fände es sich wirklich so, so wäre dieses eine überraschende Bestättigung der vorliegenden Theorie. In den mir gegenwärtig zu Gebote stehenden Werken habe ich hierüber, und dass diese Anomalie in eine Periode eingeschlossen sey, nichts erwähnt gefunden.

§. 11.

Bevor *Olauf Roemer* uns die Geschwindigkeit des Lichtes kennen lehrte und selbst noch viele Jahre nach ihm hielt man an der Meinung fest, dass keine Bewegung am Himmel und auf Erden mit jener des Lichtes in irgend einen Vergleich kommen könne und bei einer Gesichtswahrnehmung einen auch noch so geringen Einfluss auf dieselbe auszuüben vermögen werde. Die scharfsinnige Erklärung des Aberrations-Phänomens, diesem Wahne entgegentretend, verdankte es ganz der unwiderstehlichen Kraft der Wahrheit ihrer Lehre, wenn sie gleichwohl in nicht gar langer Zeit sich allgemeine Anerkennung erwarb. Ist aber eine Geschwindigkeit von 4·7 Meilen hinreichend, die Richtung des Lichtstrahls um 20″ abzulenken, warum sollte nicht eine nachweisbar ungleich grössere eine Aenderung in Farbe und Intensität des Lichtes bewirken? Nichts kann einen Forscher hindern, sich und andern eine solche Frage vorzulegen und in deren Beantwortung sich zu versuchen. Ob uns die dermalen vorliegenden Beobachtungen schon in den Stand setzen werden, diese Frage zu einer definitiven Beantwortung zu

hours suddenly become visible and remain so for some time before gradually fading until they totally disapear within a few years.

8. In the same way, this explains why the so-called new and lost stars, running through all the colours of the rainbow, finally disappear with a copper-red light. Most probably, no small number of those stars which we take for unmoving and unchanging have undergone a similar colour and light change, as indeed is without doubt in reference to Sirius.

Fig. 8

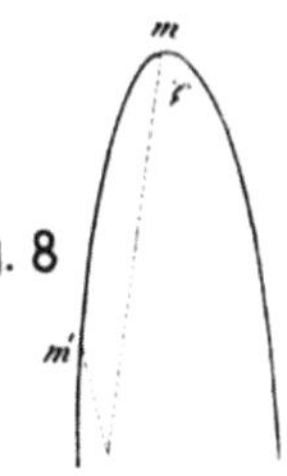

9. At last the anomalies which are observed in various periodic changing stars can most probably be expained by the movement of our Earth. So, for example, the star Mira at the neck of Cetus sometimes shows a period of light-change of 328 ½ days, sometimes again one of 335 ½ days, thus a difference of 7 days. Since the orbit of our Earth takes 365 ¼ days, so the Earth is each year under a different sign when this star attains its greatest brightness, and the direction of its movement towards or away from this star is thus different each year. But since the movement of the Earth must undoubtedly exert an influence on the star entering the phase of its greatest brightness, so will this happen somewhat earlier at one time and so much later at another. A difference in speed of 43.2 miles would delay or advance this greatest brightness by 7 whole days. If this be correct, it must be possible to prove the periodicity of about 12 years for this apparent anomaly of the star Mira, and, if it were found to be truly so, then this would be a supris-ing confirmation of the theory put forward here. In the works at present available to me I have found no mention of this, nor also that this anomaly is locked into a periodicity.

§ 11.

Before *Olauf Roemer* taught us the speed of light and even many years after him, one was of the firm opinion that no movement in heaven or on Earth could come into any way in comparison with that of light and that not even personal observation could have the slightest effect on this belief. The perspicacious explanation of the phenonenom of aberration, standing against this delusion, is wholly indebted to the irresistable strength of the truth in its teaching for the fact that it has achieved general recognition within a short time. But if a speed of 21.6 miles is sufficient to divert the direction of a beam of light by 20″, then why should not a demonstrably greater one cause a change in the colour and intensity of the light? Nothing can prevent a researcher from considering such a question and attempting to find its answer. Whether the observations available to us from those days are already

bringen uud dieser Theorie den Stempel einer apodiktischen Gewissheit aufzudrücken, will ich der Entscheidung der eigentlichen Sachkenner anheimstellen. So viel indessen scheint gewiss, dass, das hier durchgeführte Raisonnement als richtig vorausgesetzt, hiermit einer Theorie eine Grundlage gegeben ist, von welcher die berühmte *Bradley*'sche Aberrations-Lehre, da sich diese nur allein auf die Richtung, jene aber auch noch überdiess auf die Farbe und Intensität des Lichtstrahls bezieht, nur als ein integrirender Theil derselben anzusehen ist, und es ist fast für gewiss anzunehmen, dass dieselbe in nicht ferner Zukunft den Astronomen ein willkommenes Mittel darbieten dürfte, die Bewegungen und Entfernungen selbst solcher Gestirne zu bestimmen, welche wegen ihrer unermesslichen Entfernungen von uns und der damit zusammenhängenden Kleinheit der paralaktischen Winkel bis zu gegenwärtigem Augenblicke kaum die Hoffnung zu solchen Messungen und Bestimmungen darboten. —

sufficient to provide a definitive answer to this question and to affix the seal of an apodictic certainty upon this theory, I will leave to the true experts to decide. So much of this seems certain that, accepting the *raisonnement* set out here as being correct, a theory is herewith given a foundation on which *Bradley's* famous teachings on aberration, since these are concerned solely with the direction but not the colour and intensity of light, can be regarded only as an integral part thereof, and it is almost to be accepted with certainty that this will in the not too distant future offer astronomers a welcome means to determine the movements and distances of such stars which, because of their unmeasurable distances from us and the consequent smallness of the parallactic angles, until this moment hardly presented the hope of such measurements and determinations. –

Fig. 1

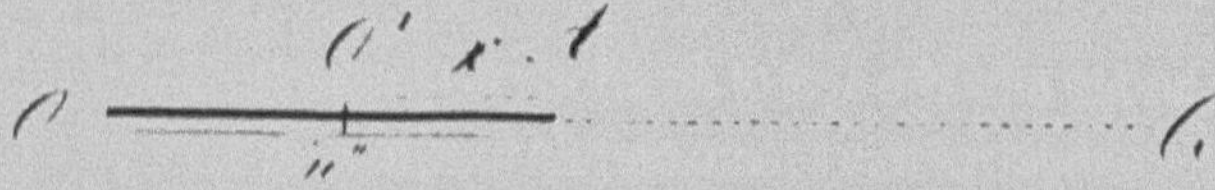

Fig. 2

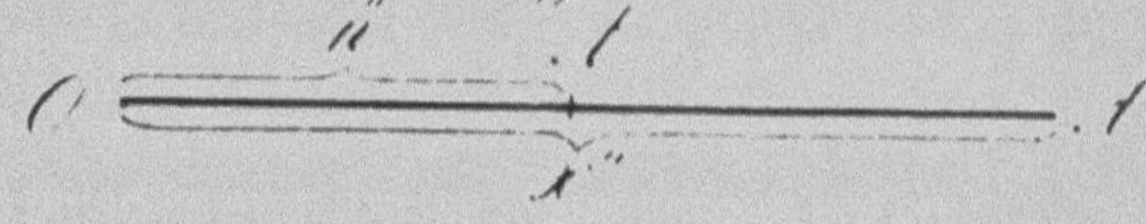

Fig. 3

Fig. 4

Fig. 5

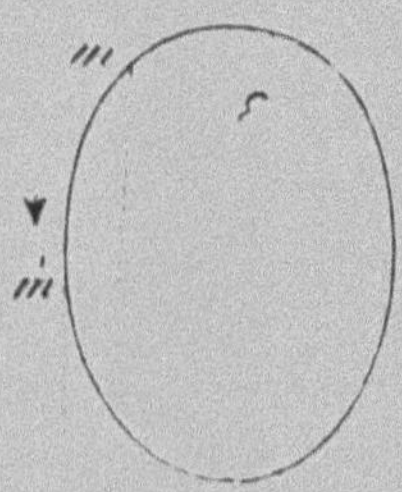

Fig. 6

Fig. 7

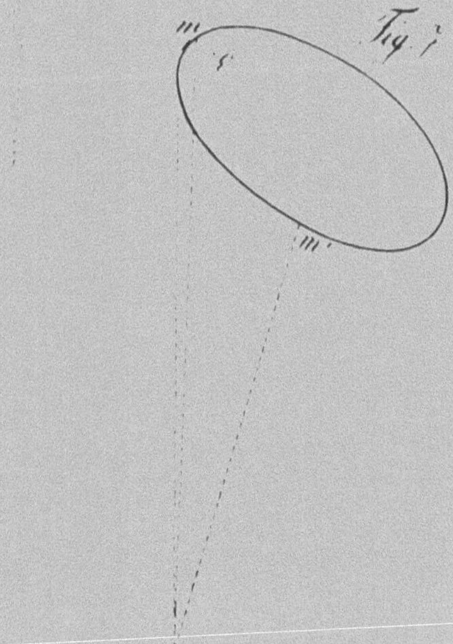

Fig. 8

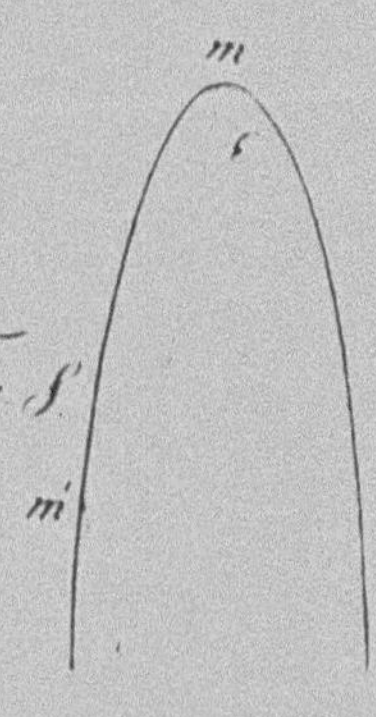

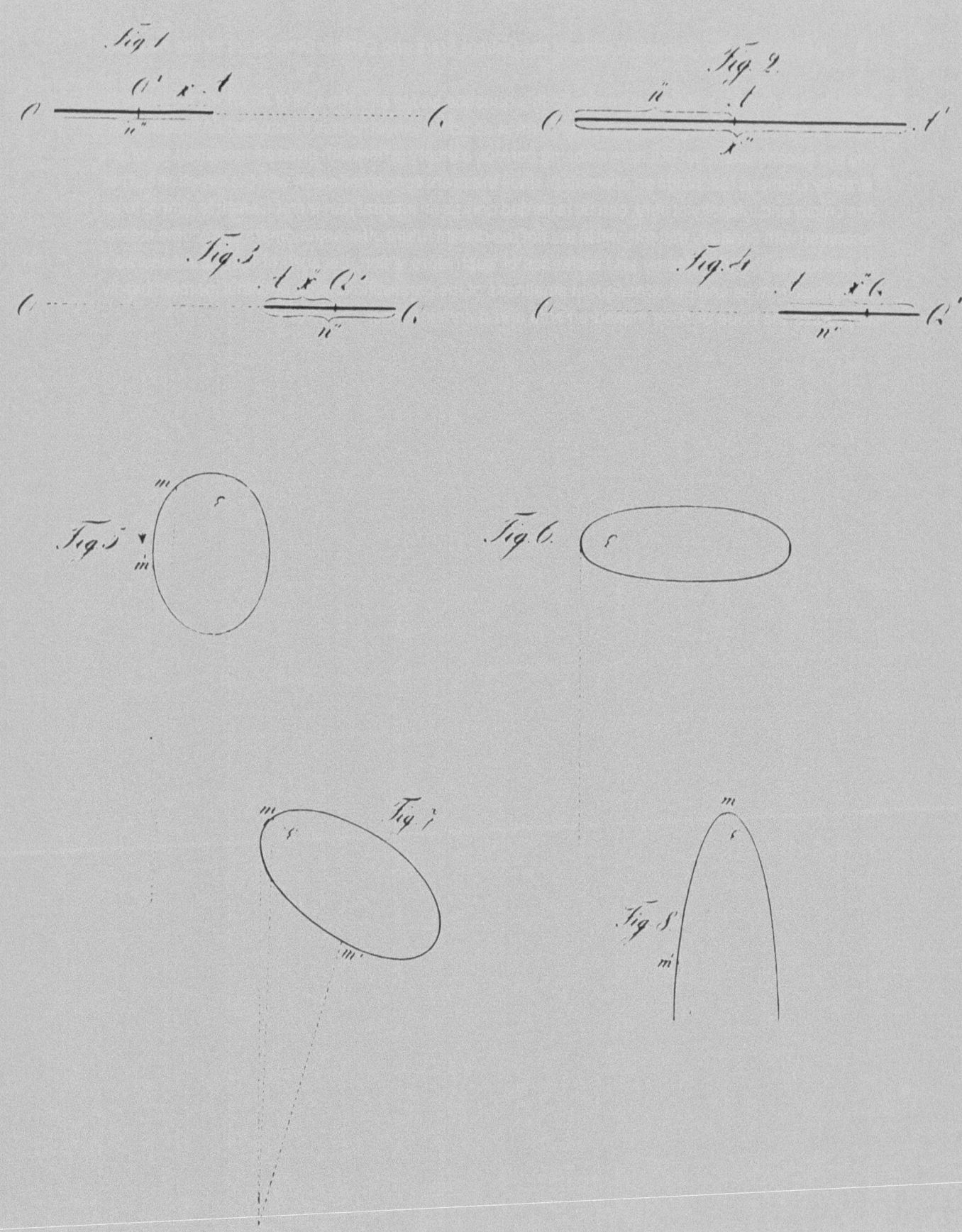

Index

FSC
www.fsc.org
MIX
Papier aus verantwortungsvollen Quellen
Paper from responsible sources
FSC® C105338

If you have any concerns about our products,
you can contact us on
ProductSafety@springernature.com

In case Publisher is established outside the EU,
the EU authorized representative is:
Springer Nature Customer Service Center GmbH
Europaplatz 3, 69115 Heidelberg, Germany

Printed by Libri Plureos GmbH
in Hamburg, Germany